Antidepressants and Social Anxiety

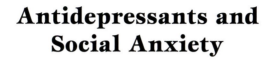

A Pill for Shyness?

ANTIDEPRESSANTS

ANTIDEPRESSANTS

Antidepressants and Social Anxiety

A Pill for Shyness?

by Joyce Libal

Mason Crest Publishers

Philadelphia

Mason Crest Publishers Inc.
370 Reed Road
Broomall, Pennsylvania 19008
(866) MCP-BOOK (toll free)

First printing
1 2 3 4 5 6 7 8 9 10

Library of Congress Cataloging-in-Publication Data

Libal, Joyce.
  Antidepressants and social anxiety : a pill for shyness? / by Joyce Libal.
    p. cm. — (Antidepressants)
  Includes bibliographical references and index.
  ISBN 1-4222-0098-1   ISBN 1-4222-0094-9 (series)
  1. Antidepressants—Juvenile literature. 2. Social phobia—Juvenile lit-
erature. I. Title. II. Series.
  RM332.L53 2007
  615'.78—dc22
                          2006005699

Interior design by MK Bassett-Harvey.
Interiors produced by Harding House Publishing Service, Inc.
www.hardinghousepages.com.
Cover design by Peter Culatta.
Printed in the Hashemite Kingdom of Jordan.

Contents

Introduction

by Andrew M. Kleiman, M.D.

From ancient Greece through the twenty-first century, the experience of sadness and depression is one of the many that define humanity. As long as human beings have felt emotions, they have endured depression. Experienced by people from every race, socioeconomic class, age group, and culture, depression is an emotional and physical experience that millions of people suffer each day. Despite being described in literature and music; examined by countless scientists, philosophers, and thinkers; and studied and treated for centuries, depression continues to remain as complex and mysterious as ever.

In today's Western culture, hearing about depression and treatments for depression is common. Adolescents in particular are bombarded with information, warnings, recommendations, and suggestions. It is critical that adolescents and young people have an understanding of depression and its impact on an individual's psychological and physical health, as well as the treatment options available to help those who suffer from depression.

Why? Because depression can lead to poor school performance, isolation from family and friends, alcohol and drug abuse, and even suicide. This doesn't have to be the case, since many useful and promising treatments exist to relieve the suffering of those with depression. Treatments for depression may also pose certain risks, however.

Since the beginning of civilization, people have been trying to alleviate the suffering of those with depression. Modern-day medicine and psychology have taken the understanding and treatment of depression to new heights. Despite their shortcomings, these treatments have helped millions and millions of people lead happier, more fulfilling and prosperous lives that would not be possible in generations past. These treatments, however, have their own risks, and for some people, may not be effective at all. Much work in neuroscience, medicine, and psychology needs to be done in the years to come.

Many adolescents experience depression, and this book series will help young people to recognize depression both in themselves and in those around them. It will give them the basic understanding of the history of depression and the various treatments that have been used to combat depression over the years. The books will also provide a basic scientific understanding of depression, and the many biological, psychological, and alternative treatments available to someone suffering from depression today.

Each person's brain and biology, life experiences, thoughts, and day-to-day situations are unique. Similarly, each individual experiences depression and sadness in a unique way. Each adolescent suffering from depression thus requires a distinct, individual treatment plan that best suits his or her needs. This series promises to be a vital resource for helping young people recognize and understand depression, and make informed and thoughtful decisions regarding treatment.

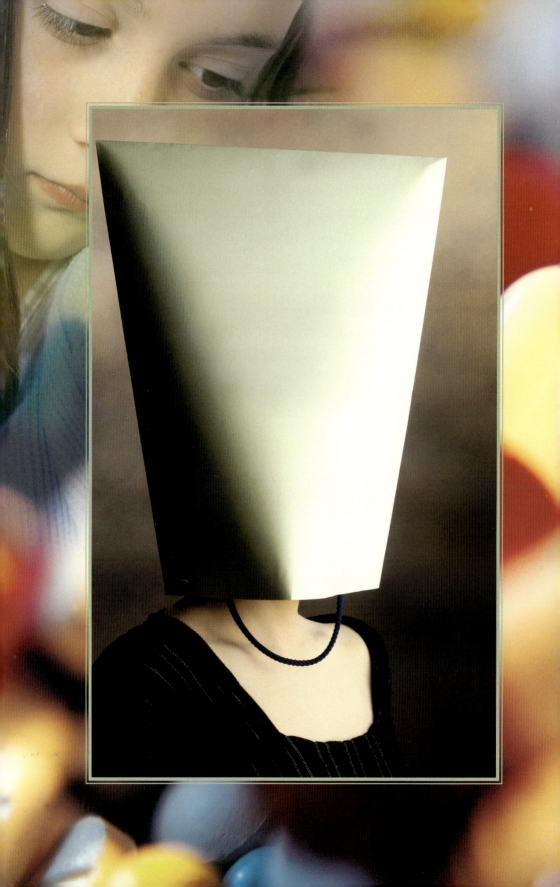

Chapter 1

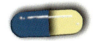

What Is Social Anxiety?

Hello World,

I s anyone out there like me? I've been shy all my life, and it's causing some real problems. I never had many friends, but now, at age nineteen, I feel like I'm totally alone. It's driving me crazy. It seems like I spend more time (way more time) talking to myself in my head every day than I've spent talking to other people my whole life. Okay, that might be an exaggeration, but even the simplest things other people do every day (things they love to do) practically paralyze me with nervousness: shopping, going to parties, dating—forget about it. An invitation to any of them might sound good at first, for about a second, then I start thinking about all the ways I'll probably embarrass myself if I go: I'll pick the wrong clothes for the party and look really out of place. Everybody will see me when I walk in the door and realize I have no sense of style. Because I'm so nervous I might get clumsy. No one will want to talk to me, and if anyone does, I'll say something stupid. I know for sure I'll blush because I'm the biggest blusher in the world. Sometimes my face gets so hot I feel like I could faint from embarrassment. If the floor could open and swallow me forever at times like that, I'd go willingly. I can't stand it anymore. I don't want to be like this. Please don't think I'm conceited, but I do have some talents, and I wish I could share them with others. I write music and I have a good voice. Now I'm about to announce my biggest secret to the whole World Wide Web: Part of me would love to try out for *American Idol*. If the people who know me ever heard that, I'm sure they'd be shocked and get a big laugh out of it. Anyway, I'm certainly too terrified to ever do anything like that. I don't want to make a fool of myself in front of millions of people. My mom says I'm my own worst enemy because I stop myself from doing so many things, but I can't get rid of the negative thoughts in my head. I know it isn't rational to be so worried about what other people think of me, but I can't stop. Can anybody out there relate to any of this? Or am I the only weird and pathetic one?

Thanks for listening,
Scared All the Time

What's Wrong with Being Shy?

Think about the emotions this person described in her blog: shyness, anxiety, fear. How would you define each of them? Perhaps some of these definitions come to mind:

Shyness: modesty; an unassuming, reserved, humble, retiring, bashful, timid, unassertive, self-conscious, awkward, submissive attitude

Anxiety: uneasiness, apprehension, nervousness, agitation, feeling of dread or impending doom, intense worry caused by not being able to control events that are about to take place

Fear: trepidation, extreme anxiety caused by imminent danger, alarm, panic, terror

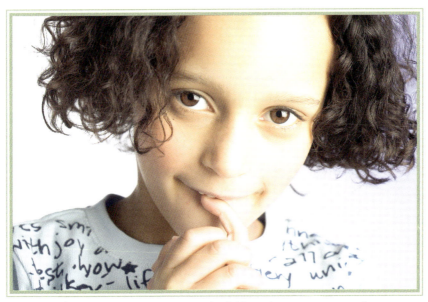

Shyness is a common childhood experience that most people outgrow enough to function in the work world and in social situations.

Shyness, anxiety, and fear are not the same things, and they're not necessarily bad things. Many admirable qualities are associated with being shy. There's also nothing wrong with feeling anxious in certain situations. While taking a test or performing at a recital, some level of this emotion is expected. Anxiety can be a motivator that encourages us to complete tasks and prepare properly for upcoming events. And there's a proper time to be fearful—in dangerous situations. But severe shyness can cause anxiety, and extreme anxiety can lead to a type of fear that is unnecessary. When shyness, anxiety, and fear are carried to their extremes, and when these extremes become nearly constant, they can have negative health consequences. They can also interfere with common aspects of living one's life.

What's Wrong with Scared All the Time?

Millions of people use adjectives like shy, *introverted*, quiet, or *introspective* to describe themselves, and the world benefits from having people with these personality traits. In some cultures, these are considered to be among the most sought-after virtues. But Scared All the Time is not simply shy. She is experiencing a level of social anxiety that is debilitating and sometimes overpowering. This type of anxiety cuts across race and social class, placing constant restraints on the lives of those who experience it on a regular basis.

Medical professionals use a book called the *Diagnostic and Statistical Manual of Mental Disorders, Fourth Edition* (DSM-IV) to determine when social anxiety (also called social

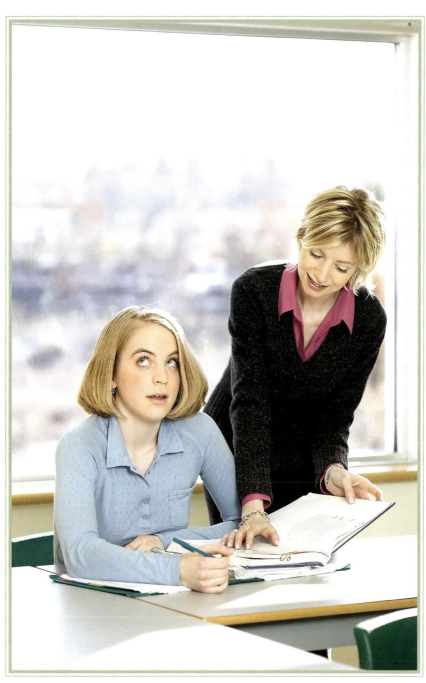

Everyone feels anxious in certain situations—
like being called on by a teacher.

phobia) is so severe that it is classified as a mental disorder. People with this disorder fear social situations because they are worried about doing something humiliating. They are self-conscious about being evaluated and judged, and these feelings bring on tremendous anxiety. People with social anxiety disorder are easily embarrassed, and they feel inadequate

What's a Phobia?

Many medical professionals prefer the term social anxiety to social phobia because they think the word "phobia" is difficult for some people to understand and is too narrow in scope to adequately describe social anxiety disorder. "Phobia" means a powerful and irrational fear. Many people who do not have social phobia experience phobias to other things. Maybe you have one of the dozens of common phobias that exist; a few are listed here:

aichmophobia = fear of needles or other pointy objects
arachnophobia = fear of spiders
bibliophobia = fear of books
claustrophobia = fear of confined spaces
coulrophobia = fear of clowns
decidophobia = fear of making decisions
hemophobia = fear of blood
hypengyophobia = fear of responsibility
iatrophobia = fear of going to the doctor's
suriphobia = fear of mice

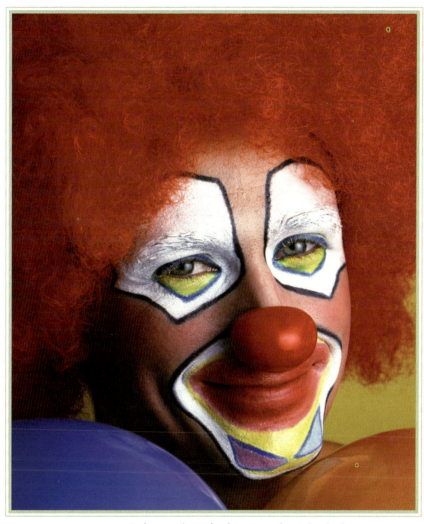

A person with coulrophobia is afraid of clowns.

and ill equipped to deal with the social aspects of everyday life. Approximately 13 percent of the population is believed to have this disorder.

The term "generalized" is sometimes used to describe the type of social anxiety that involves most community

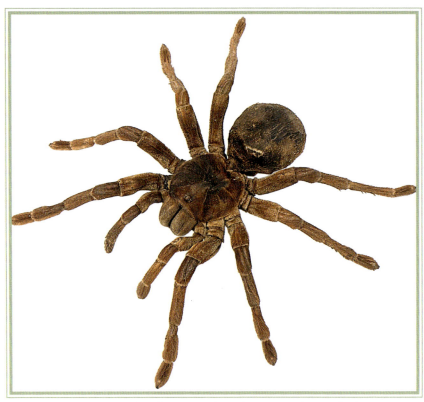

A person who fears spiders has arachnophobia,
a phobia shared by many Westerners.

situations, as was described by Scared All the Time. Sometimes people can easily engage in the majority of social interactions but have intense anxiety in just one or two specific areas. For example, many people fear making a formal presentation before a large group. Fewer people fear writing in public, like signing a credit slip when shopping or filling out a form at a doctor's office. Some people find it impossible to urinate in public restrooms (often called shy bladder syndrome).

All of these occurrences describe social anxieties. Situations like these are sometimes called "performance" phobias, "specific" phobias, or "discreet" phobias. Other types of specific social anxieties include but are not limited to: fear of reading aloud in front of others, fear of initiating conversations, fear of making phone calls in public places, and fear of eating in front of other people. Approximately one-fourth of those with social anxiety disorder have the specific form; the remainder suffers with the more devastating generalized type.

Symptoms

Scared All the Time describes psychological and physical symptoms that are typical of social anxiety disorder: consistent negative thoughts in anticipation of social situations, intense fear of being humiliated in front of other people, realization that these negative thoughts and fears are irrational, avoidance of social situations, severe blushing, and extreme loneliness. Like blushing, other physical symptoms may be present when people with this disorder are confronted with the situations that stimulate their anxiety. Examples include profuse sweating, stomachaches, diarrhea, headaches, jitteriness, vomiting, and accelerated heartbeat.

Sometimes people have medical conditions that cause shaking (as in Parkinson's disease), stuttering, cardiac problems, or other physical symptoms that could cause embarrassment in public situations. Anxiety caused by medical conditions does not meet the criteria for a diagnosis of social anxiety disorder.

Youth and Social Anxiety Disorder

If an individual is going to develop social anxiety disorder, it usually happens before the person reaches her mid-twenties; typically, it begins in the teen years. Younger children who are consistently withdrawn and fearful in new situations may have a tendency to develop social anxiety disorder. Children with these tendencies experience anxiety when engaged in social interactions (or when anticipating these events) with their peers rather than just having anxiety when interacting with adults, and they might not recognize their fear as unreasonable in the way adults do. According to the DSM-IV, children might express this anxiety by "crying, tantrums, freezing, or shrinking from social situations with unfamiliar people." Clinging to parents or even **selective mutism** are other possible symptoms. Social anxiety must last for more than six months in individuals under the age of eighteen in order to be classified as social anxiety disorder.

The Positive Side of Fear

Sometimes a person's safety can depend on recognition of a situation as dangerous. In these cases, anxiety and fear cause the person to react in a way that may even save his life. When faced with a life-threatening situation, a person experiences a rush of adrenaline (also called epinephrine) and other hormones; he then quickly makes the decision to stay and fight or flee the situation. This is known as the "fight-or-flight" response, and over centuries it has been necessary to the survival of the human species.

Diagnostic Criteria for Social Anxiety/Social Phobia

• The individual has a marked and persistent fear of one or more social or performance situations in which the person is exposed to unfamiliar people or to possible scrutiny by others. The individual fears that he or she will act in a way (or show anxiety symptoms) that will be humiliating or embarrassing.

• Exposure to the feared social situation almost invariably provokes anxiety, which may take the form of a situationally bound or situationally predisposed panic attack.

• The person recognizes that the fear is excessive or unreasonable.

• The feared social or performance situations are avoided or else are endured with intense anxiety or distress.

• The avoidance, anxious anticipation, or distress in the feared social or performance situation(s) interferes significantly with the person's normal routine, occupational (academic) functioning, or social activities or relationships, or there is marked distress about having the phobia.

• The fear or avoidance is not due to direct physiological effects of a substance (such as a drug of abuse or a medication) or to a general medical condition and is not better accounted for by another mental disorder.

Adapted from the Diagnostic and Statistical Manual of Mental Disorders-IV-Text Revision

An increased heart rate is among the physiological responses that take place during this "adrenaline rush." Sweating, another response, is a way for the body to regulate its temperature during this fear-causing event. Automatic responses like these are gen-

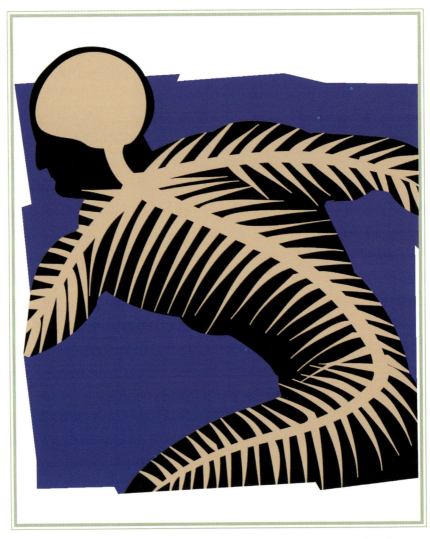

Anxiety affects your entire nervous system, which in turn causes a wide range of physical effects.

erated by the "sympathetic nervous system," and they assist the body as it either fights or flees.

Unfortunately, many people with social anxiety disorder feel this level of stress and fear at unrealistic times—in social situations—and it can happen on a daily basis. For them, automatic responses like sweating can become a source of embarrassment. Often people with this disorder react by avoiding the situations that cause these extreme emotions.

People also have a "parasympathetic nervous system" that helps keep the sympathetic nervous system in control and assists the body in returning to normal when danger has passed. The parasympathetic nervous system can have another effect as well. If you have ever been in a car accident or other dangerous situation, you may have felt like the world was moving in slow motion. That feeling was caused by the parasympathetic nervous system. When someone talks about being "paralyzed with fear," it is this system that is causing the temporary paralysis. The parasympathetic nervous system kicks in automatically when both fighting and fleeing are impossible, and it may also have a role in social anxiety disorder.

Avoidance Tactics

Many shy individuals function perfectly well in the world. While they may be somewhat uncomfortable in certain social situations, they are not filled with dread at the thought of interacting with people and do not work to actively avoid these occasions. Shy people with social anxiety disorder, on the other hand, often go to great lengths to avoid stressful social situations. They may deprive themselves of extracurricular activities such as band and sports, shun certain dating situations, select a college based on fear of moving away from home or leaving friends, avoid employment and remain financially tied to their parents, or accept a job that is below their ambitions and abilities because they fear interpersonal

Avoidant Behaviors

Sometimes people with social anxiety disorder do not avoid social situations but use avoidant methods to cope with them. For example, they might:

• hold objects to avoid trembling.

• resist making eye contact with others.

• give only short answers to questions because they fear fumbling over words or stuttering.

• speak very quickly, avoiding pauses because they fear their mind will "go blank" during a pause.

• leave social gatherings early to minimize interpersonal contacts.

Avoidant behaviors prevent an individual from seeing for himself that his fears are unjustified. Also, many of these behaviors may be interpreted negatively by witnesses, thus preventing the person with social anxiety disorder from experiencing the kind of positive feedback that could make it easier to face social situations in the future.

actions that would be required in other employment positions. Under circumstances like these, it is in the best interest of people with social anxiety disorder to take steps to bring these emotions and actions under control.

Some medical professionals do not treat this disorder seriously. They see shyness as a common personality trait and social anxiety as a normal part of life. It is true that shyness is not a "weakness," and we certainly should not be trying to stamp it out. However, it is critical to distinguish between the kind of shyness and anxiety that are natural and manageable, and social anxiety disorder. Individuals with this disorder can improve their lives immeasurably by seeking help from health-care professionals trained to recognize and treat this condition. Without proper diagnosis and treatment, they are likely to view their lives through the lens of social anxiety, making critical decisions concerning education, employment, and even personal relationships based on fear. Additionally, without treatment they are at high risk for using alcohol or drugs to cope with their disorder and of sinking into deepening depression.

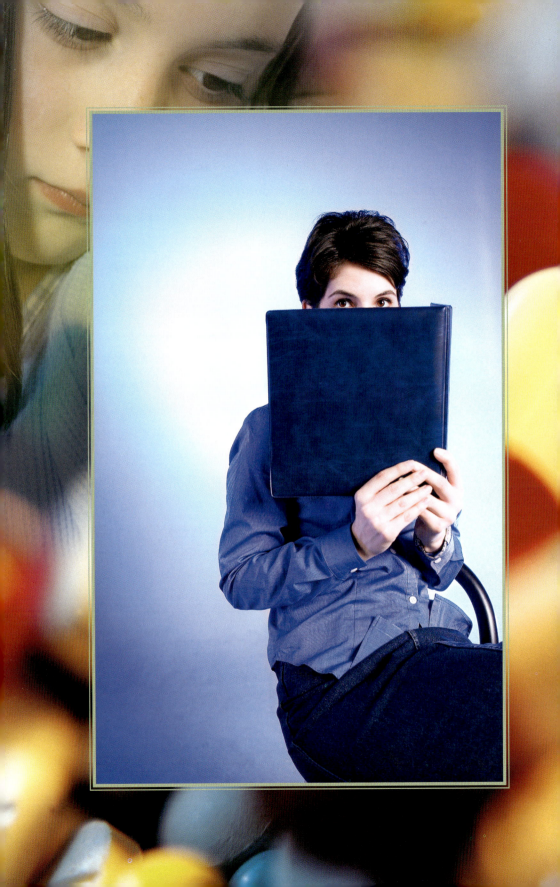

Chapter 2

Diagnosis and Misdiagnosis

Dear Scared All the Time,

Your posting really hit home with me. Like you, I don't know why I'm so concerned about what other people think of me, but it's been this way as long as I can remember. I have one really vivid memory that goes back to when I was nine. Dad took Mom and me to McDonald's. We were standing in line, and I whispered my order to Dad so he could tell it to the teenager at the counter. Mom thought it would be good for me to speak directly to the person at the counter rather than relying on Dad for that. I was too shy and nervous to do it, so we had a bit of a scene over the whole thing with her eventually giving in and Dad placing my order. Anyway, when it was over I turned to walk to a booth and noticed three girls from my class. They were in line behind us, had witnessed the entire thing, and were poking each other and giggling; I was mortified! Later, when we were eating, I glanced over

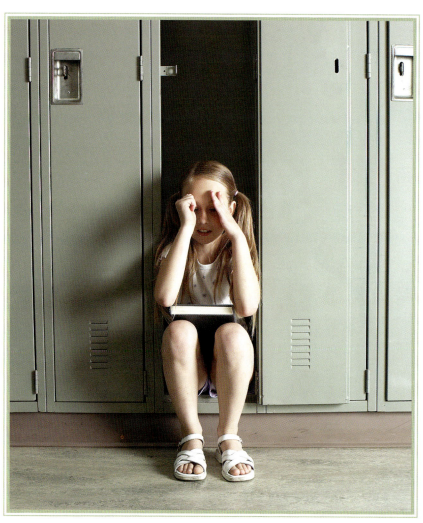

Many young people feel anxious in certain school situations.

to their table and saw them looking at me. I could barely touch another bite. Then on Monday (our first day back at school after the McDonald's incident), the teacher called on me to work a math problem at the board; I couldn't believe my bad luck. I heard giggling as I walked to the front of the class. My hand started to tremble when I picked up the chalk. My mind went blank as numbers began to swim on the other side of my eyes. Luckily, I didn't start openly sobbing. Eventually the answer came to me, but it took much longer than it should have, and I felt like the dumbest kid on the planet. It seemed like an eternity before I got back to my seat, and when I glanced up at the board, my answer looked shaky, like the numbers had been written by a kindergartner. I felt so ashamed. I spent the rest of the day (maybe the week) reliving the whole, horrible thing. I've had lots of similar incidents since then. I'm fourteen now, and my self-esteem has been in the toilet since at least the fourth grade. I can't help but notice other kids having fun at school—going to dances, playing sports, just hanging out together. I wish I could be more like them, but that seems impossible. I don't know what to do about all of this. I know I'll never be the most popular kid in school, but I wish I could be normal.

Thanks for your posting. It's nice to have someone to talk to.

—Why me?

What Causes Social Anxiety?

Some people with social anxiety disorder remember a single traumatic event they believe triggered their condition; others have no such memory. Even those who have such a memory might be incorrect about it actually having caused their disorder.

Childhood Risk Factors

Having these factors does not mean you will develop social anxiety disorder, but the risk of doing so may be increased.

• being the firstborn male in a family

• having a parent or sibling with social anxiety disorder

• extended separation from parents

• being a victim of sexual abuse

• academic failure during primary school

• being in a family that moves to new residences more than three times

• running away from home and family

• not having a close relationship with an adult

• involvement with the criminal justice system

• dropping out of high school

(Compiled from several studies.)

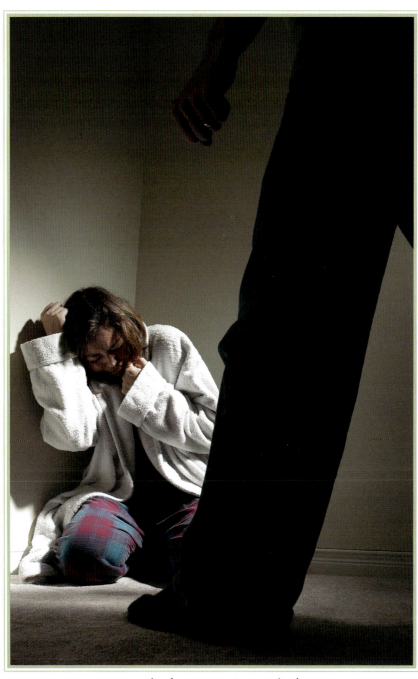

A person who has experienced abuse is at risk for developing an anxiety disorder.

Scientists do not know the exact reasons why some people develop social anxiety disorder, and research into this is ongoing. Genetic factors influence both the biology and chemistry of the brain. Neurotransmitters (various chemicals released by nerve endings in the brain) most likely play a role. (More about how neurotransmitters work in the brain appears in chapter 3.) The amount of serotonin, dopamine, norepinephrine (also called noradrenaline), and other neurotransmitters available in an individual's brain can be influenced by genetics.

Other factors in social anxiety disorder may also be related to genetic background. **Peripheral** benzodiazepine receptors (explained further in chapter 3) do not occur only in the brain; instead, they are located throughout the body. These receptors play a role in regulating hormones that cause symptoms related to stress. Some people with anxiety disorders might have abnormal levels of these receptors.

Both genetics and environment are probably responsible for social anxiety disorder. A tendency toward many different psychiatric disorders can be inherited, but environment (such as how a child is parented, her experiences in peer groups or lack of peer-group experiences, being a victim of bullying or traumatic events, and negative classroom situations) can also play an important role in their development.

Diagnosis

Men are most likely to seek treatment for social anxiety disorder, but just as many women have the condition. Most people

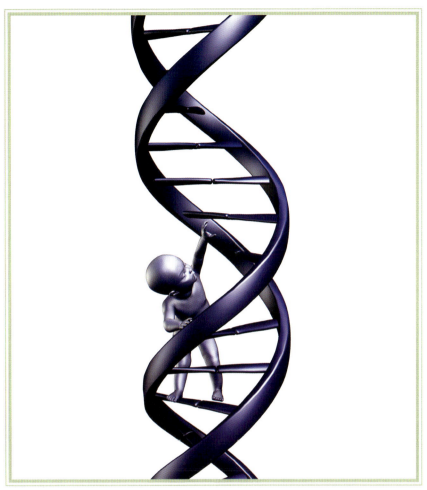

Social anxiety may be caused by environment—and by the genetic tendencies passed along through the generations.

struggle through it alone or with the support of close family members and never seek treatment. This can be devastating for those with the generalized form of the condition, but even people with specific forms can benefit from treatment. The first step is to seek a proper diagnosis. This involves meeting with a medical doctor, psychologist, social worker, or psychiatrist who is knowledgeable about the disorder. The first meeting will involve many questions and possibly some tests aimed at assessing the individual's physical and mental states.

Misdiagnosis

Because treatment for different psychiatric disorders varies, correct diagnosis is necessary to assure proper medical care. Sometimes social anxiety disorder is present along with another psychiatric disorder. Medical practitioners use the term "comorbidity" to describe this. Even when additional psychiatric conditions are not present, similarities between social anxiety disorder and certain other disorders can make correct diagnosis difficult. Some of these disorders are briefly described here.

Panic Disorder

People with panic disorder often experience the same physical symptoms as those with social anxiety disorder, but the cause of the symptoms and the individual's feelings about them differ. With panic disorder, people may have symptoms when no one else is present. In other words, their panic attack is usually not brought on by a social situation. Additionally, individuals often fear they will die because of the severity of their attack; conversely, those with social anxiety disorder fear the humiliation they'll suffer because of having attack symptoms in front of other people. It's possible for a person with social anxiety disorder to also have panic disorder, but these are

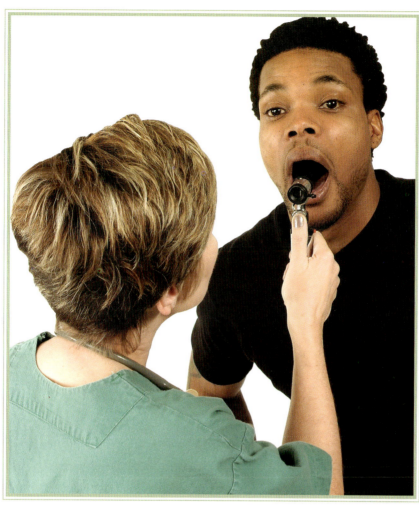

If you consult your doctor about social anxiety, the first visit will likely involve a general examination, to rule out any physical reasons for your feelings.

separate disorders with separate causes. Some different parts of the brain (including different chemicals and receptors) are involved in the two disorders.

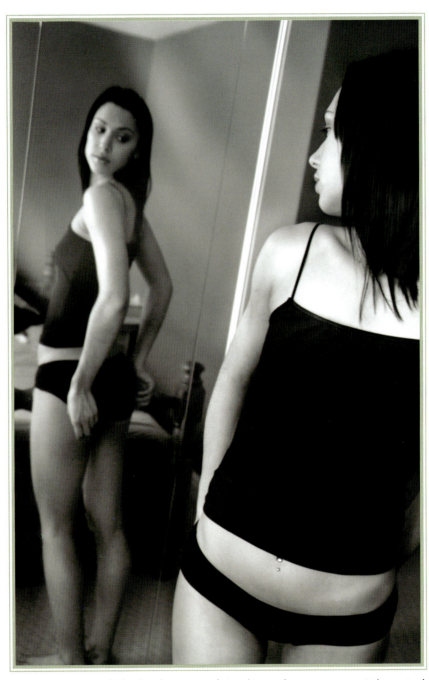

A person with body dysmorphic disorder may avoid social situations because she hates what she sees in the mirror.

Avoidant Personality Disorder

As the name implies, individuals with this condition "avoid" social situations. Like those with social anxiety disorder, they fear doing anything embarrassing in front of others and genuinely believe they are unworthy of social companionship. Whereas people with social anxiety disorder realize their feelings are unrealistic, those with avoidant personality disorder don't believe there is anything inaccurate about their thinking and generally do not seek help to change it.

Agoraphobia

This disorder can also develop as a reaction to panic attacks. Sometimes people who experience these attacks become so fearful of having them in a place where they cannot easily escape that they become homebound. Even if they can force themselves to leave their house or apartment, they often allow themselves to visit only a limited number of places (just their home and office, for example, or their home and the home of a trusted relative).

Body Dysmorphic Disorder

People with body dysmorphic disorder may avoid social settings because they're convinced something about their physical appearance is hideous, and they don't want to have it observed by others. This reason for avoiding social interaction is different from that of social anxiety disorder.

Depression

Living with social anxiety disorder often leads to depression. As depression escalates, individuals may even begin to have thoughts of suicide. The potentially fatal nature of depression makes ***intervention*** especially important in these cases. Depression and social anxiety disorder are separate illnesses, however, and even though they can be comorbid, they usually need to each be specifically addressed during treatment.

Social Anxiety Self-Test

If you answer yes to the following questions, it is important to discuss these feelings with your parents and family doctor.

- *Do you experience anxiety and fear at the thought of being in a social situation where other people could judge you?*

- *Do you worry excessively about humiliating yourself in front of others?*

- *Are you very concerned that others will notice physical signs of your anxiety such as sweating, trembling, or blushing?*

- *Do you think your social fears are unreasonable or excessive?*

- *Does the feared social situation ever cause you to experience panic attacks, meaning physical symptoms such as sweating, trembling, dizziness, chest pain, or racing or pounding heart, shortness of breath, choking sensations, nausea or stomachaches, or does it make you feel wobbly or "detached" from yourself?*

- *Do you find excuses to avoid social situations?*

- *Does social anxiety interfere with the way you want to live your life?*

Generalized Anxiety Disorder

People with social anxiety often have a condition called generalized anxiety disorder (GAD) as well. This means they also experience anxiety in other situations beside social ones. Although all people feel worried or anxious sometimes, this disorder refers to a level of anxiety that is excessive, chronic, and typically interferes with the individual's ability to function in normal daily activities. Generalized anxiety is sometimes called "free-floating" anxiety because it is not triggered by a specific object or situation.

It is perfectly normal to have some social anxiety before a big dance or an oral report. These feelings can even be helpful, encouraging you to think carefully and do your best. Most people (shy or not) experience these appropriate social anxieties from time to time and are able to cope with them without any form of outside treatment. Having someone to talk to can be helpful; reading self-help books might also be of assistance in overcoming unwanted shyness or controlling minor anxieties. But when someone is experiencing social anxiety to such a degree that it meets the criteria for social anxiety disorder, talking to a friend and reading books on your own are usually not adequate substitutes for professional care. Social anxiety disorder is a serious condition. It is important to evaluate a person's physical and mental health before initiating treatment, especially treatment with prescription drugs.

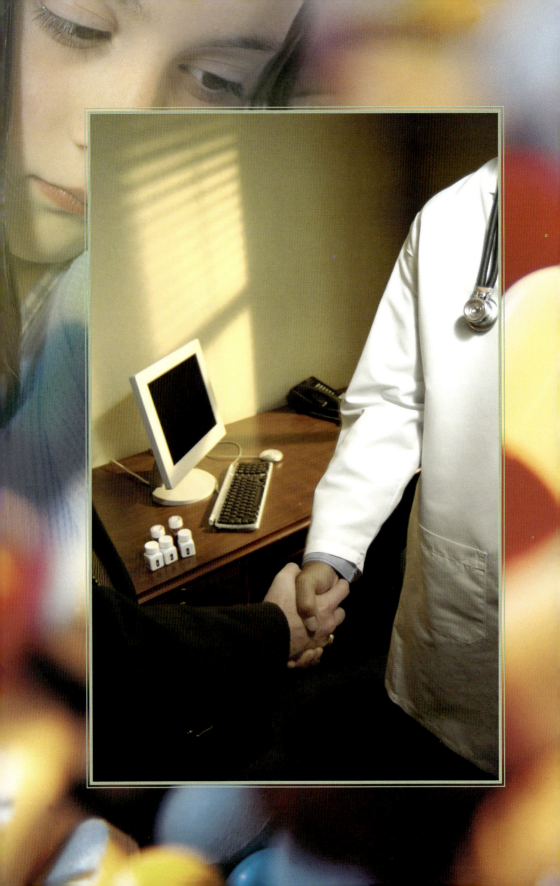

Chapter 3

Treatment Options

Dear Scared All the Time,

This may surprise you, but there's a name for what you're feeling: it's called social anxiety disorder, and you are definitely NOT alone. According to what I've read on the subject, millions of people (including me) have this condition. In fact, they say it's the third most common psychological disorder in the country. Sorry for diagnosing your condition over the Internet; only a professional can make an informed diagnosis, of course. But the things you describe sound like you took a page out of the book of my life. And guess what? I've discovered that having a "psychological disorder" doesn't have to be as bad as it sounds. I've had treatment (cognitive-behavioral therapy) that really worked, and I still attend a support group once a week. What a godsend! I've got to run, have to be at work in forty-five minutes, but I'll write again soon. Incidentally, while I'm at work today, I'll be giving a presentation to our company's board of directors, and I'm completely prepared to do it. Am I nervous? Of course I am, but I'm keeping it in control, keeping it real, not pre-living it and overexaggerating it in my head. In five minutes I'll be in my car singing with the radio and NOT worrying about what's going to happen when I get to the office. That would not have been possible for me a year and a half ago. Back then, I couldn't even look my supervisor in the eye. So, like I said before, I'll write again soon. In the meantime, don't give up hope. There's help out there for people like us.

—No Longer SAD (Social Anxiety Disorder)

Some Treatments Don't Work

No Longer SAD successfully conquered social anxiety disorder with a proven treatment. Various treatments are available, but some work better than others. According to factsforhealth. org, a Web site created by the Madison Institute of Medicine, relaxation therapy has been studied, shown not to be an effective treatment for social anxiety disorder, and can sometimes even *exacerbate* the condition.

While it may be useful for certain individuals, extensive *psychoanalysis* is most often not an effective treatment for social anxiety disorder. Psychoanalysis can be very helpful to

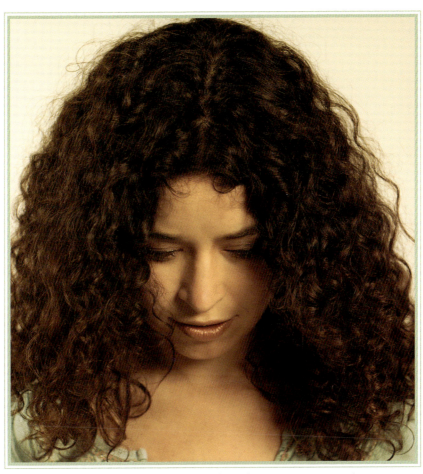

Social anxiety disorder does not respond
well to psychoanalysis.

someone with depression or certain other mental conditions, but there's rarely a reason for individuals with social anxiety disorder to spend time analyzing their past or reliving their childhood.

It is also usually not helpful to analyze one's dreams as a way of reducing the symptoms of social anxiety disorder.

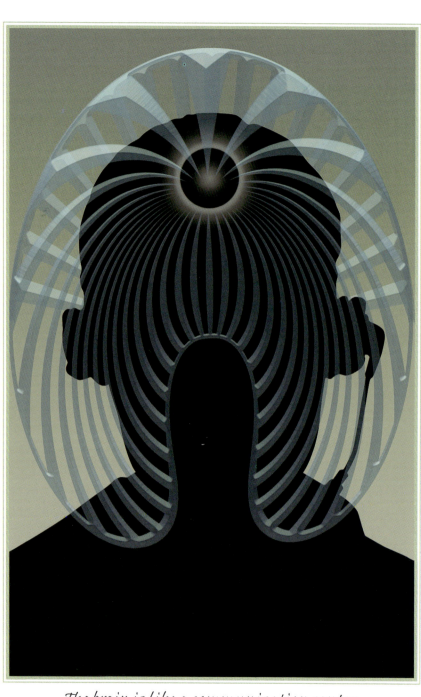

*The brain is like a communication center,
sending out messages to the entire body.*

Instead, it's best if people zero in on proven methods of eliminating irrational fears. One way of doing this is with ***cognitive***-behavioral therapy.

Cognitive-Behavioral Therapy

Many experts believe cognitive-behavioral therapy is an essential component of any successful treatment for social anxiety disorder. Basically, cognitive-behavioral therapy alters one's ***perceptions*** by providing a method of recognizing negative and irrational thought patterns that are contributing to anxiety, understanding the reasons for them, and replacing them with positive thoughts and actions. (More about cognitive-behavioral therapy is presented in chapter 5.)

Prescription Medications

To understand this treatment option, it helps to have a general knowledge of how messages are transported in the brain. Think of the brain as "communication central" for the body.

Brand Name vs. Generic Name

Talking about psychiatric drugs can be confusing, because every drug has at least two names: its "generic name" and the "brand name" that the pharmaceutical company uses to market the drug. Generic names come from the drugs' chemical structure, while drug companies use brand names to inspire public recognition and loyalty for their products.

The brain and the body are in constant communication through neurotransmitters. A neurotransmitter is a chemical compound (such as serotonin) that is released from the end of a nerve (neuron) in the brain. From there it passes across a gap (called a synapse), and then activates the receiving end (called the dendrite) of another nerve. The receiving nerve sends a neurotransmitter to another nerve, and this process is repeated. Antidepressants and antianxiety medications alter the brain's chemistry and affect this communication process. Many medical practitioners believe these prescription drugs can be effective in treating various psychiatric conditions, including social anxiety disorder.

SSRIs (Selective Serotonin Reuptake Inhibitors)

In the late 1980s, the U.S. Food and Drug Administration (FDA) began approving a classification of drugs commonly known as SSRIs. These antidepressants extend the length of time that serotonin (which is involved in mood, pain, sleep, *sensory perception*, and other activities) is available to the nerve cell receptors by preventing it from being accepted by the spaces between nerve cells (also called synaptic clefts).

Prescription drugs have both a *generic* name and a brand name. The brand name is the manufacturer's name for the drug. In the following paragraphs, the generic names for several medications appear in parentheses.

Prozac® (fluoxetine) was the first SSRI the FDA approved, but Paxil® (paroxetine) was the first one to receive official FDA

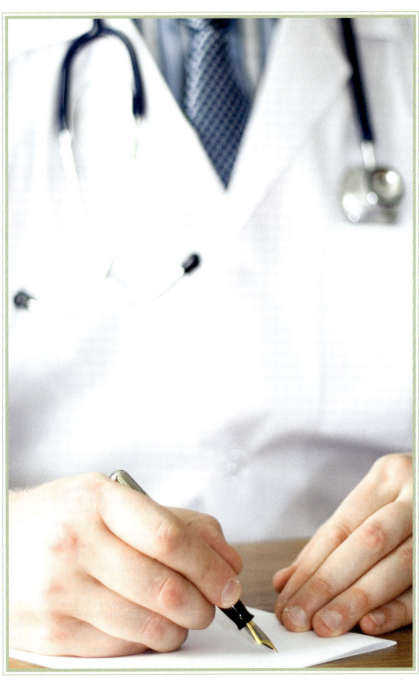

*A doctor, psychiatrist, or nurse practitioner is licensed
to prescribe an antidepressant to treat social anxiety.*

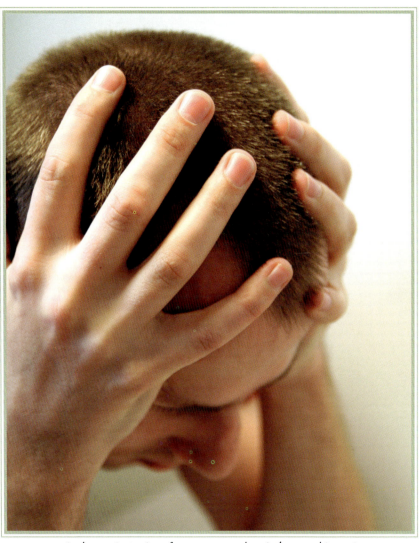

Social anxiety is often treated with medication.

approval for the treatment of social phobia. In the late 1990s, a study demonstrated improvement in more than twice as many people taking Paxil for social anxiety as those being given a placebo. Over 50 percent of those being given the drug

Drug Approval

Before a drug can be marketed in the United States, the Food and Drug Administration (FDA) must officially approve it. Today's FDA is the primary consumer protection agency in the United States. Operating under the authority given it by the government, and guided by laws established throughout the twentieth century, the FDA has created a rigorous drug approval process that verifies the safety, effectiveness, and accuracy of labeling for any drug marketed in the United States. While the United States has the FDA for the approval and regulation of drugs and medical devices, Canada has a similar organization called the Therapeutic Product Directorate (TPD). The TPD is a division of Health Canada, the Canadian government department of health. The TPD regulates drugs, medical devises, disinfectants, and sanitizers with disinfectant claims. Some of the things that the TPD monitors are quality, effectiveness, and safety. Just as the FDA must approve new drugs in the United States, the TPD must approve new drugs in Canada before those drugs can enter the market.

reported being "very much improved" or "much improved." In 2000 and 2001, the company that produces Paxil spent over $150 million promoting its use for treating anxiety. The FDA approved Zoloft® (sertraline) for treatment of social anxiety disorder next, and more recently Effexor® (venlafaxine), a serotonin and norepinephrine reuptake inhibitor (an SNRI), obtained approval for treatment of this condition.

Like Paxil, Effexor is not approved for use by anyone under the age of eighteen. Zoloft is only approved for use by children and teens for the treatment of obsessive-compulsive disorder. Doctors often treat social anxiety disorder with prescription drugs (including other antidepressants) that have not obtained FDA approval for this use. This is referred to as off-label use, and it is a legal practice. Medicines may also be prescribed for children, even when these compounds have not been proven to be safe for their use.

Those taking SSRIs for social anxiety disorder should not expect an immediate relief from anxiety. It generally takes from two to six weeks before serious improvements can be noticed.

SSRIs are powerful, mind-altering drugs. Although antidepressants can be helpful for some patients, other people report serious problems when taking them. Individuals on these medications have carried out suicides and other violent behaviors. The following testimony provides an example. It was presented at a hearing conducted by the FDA in 2004:

My name is Corey. . . . Four years ago I was diagnosed with having social anxiety disorder, and my family practitioner doctor, he prescribed Paxil [at] twenty milligrams. After about eight and a half months, I started taking forty milligrams of Paxil because it was not working at twenty milligrams. A few months after that, I went back. The same problem, it wasn't working, and he suggested I start taking a new medication called Effexor. He abruptly discontinued the Paxil and put me immediately on Effexor at seventy-five milligrams, and I was supposed to work up to three hundred milligrams. I didn't feel very well and I stayed home from school. I went back to sleep and that evening I woke up in a juvenile detention center. Unaware of what I had actually done, I asked one of the members of the juvenile detention center, and I found out that I had taken my high-powered rifle that I use for hunting to my third period class, took twenty-three of my classmates hostage and one teacher hostage. I spent fourteen months in jail, not really knowing why I had been there, not really remembering anything that I had done.

As with all medications, SSRIs can produce a number of negative side effects. The first weeks of taking one of these medications may be particularly dangerous. When a drug is discontinued or when dosages are changed are other critical times. Parents and family members should watch their loved

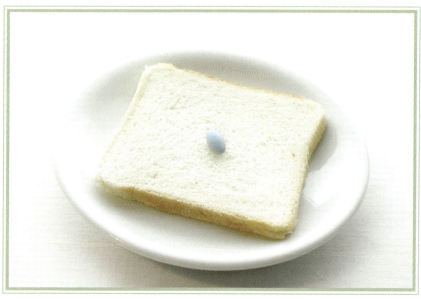

SSRIs are powerful chemicals that should not be regarded as simple answers to psychiatric disorders; like all medications, they may have side effects.

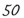

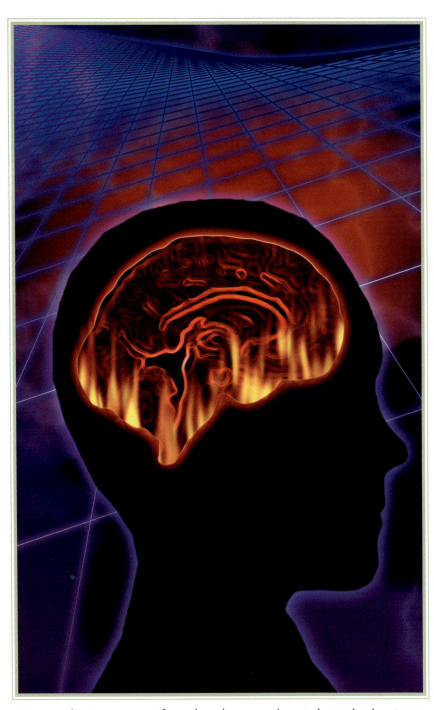

Antidepressants affect the chemicals within the brain.

one closely for changes in behavior and consult the prescribing medical practitioner immediately if they notice anything unusual. (More side effects for antidepressants are discussed in chapter 4.)

MAOIs (Monoamine Oxidase Inhibitors)

"Oxidase" refers to an **enzyme**. The neurotransmitters are "amines" because they are derived from "amino" acids. MAOIs work by interfering with the oxidase's ability to break down the amines. MAOIs affect serotonin, norepinephrine, and especially dopamine levels, allowing the brain access to a higher concentration of all three of these neurotransmitters. Drugs in this classification, especially Nardil® (phenelzine), are sometimes used to treat symptoms of social anxiety, but other classes of medications are usually preferred because of the serious dietary restrictions that are necessary when taking MAOIs and possible side effects (discussed in chapter 4). These antidepressants have been used longer than the SSRIs, but today the SSRIs are more frequently prescribed. MAOIs should never be used in combination with SSRIs, and they are not considered safe for adolescents.

RIMAs (Reversible Inhibitors of Monoamine Oxidase)

Manerix® (moclobemide), a newer antidepressant, works in the same manner as the MAOIs, but less completely. It has been less effective in treating social anxiety disorder, but it does not have the same serious dietary concerns as the MAOIs.

TCAs (Tricyclic Antidepressants)

An older tricyclic antidepressant, Tofranil® (imipramine), is also sometimes used to treat social anxiety disorder. TCAs work like SSRIs, but inhibit the reuptake of serotonin, dopamine, and norepinephrine.

Benzodiazepines

These antianxiety drugs have been readily available since the early 1960s, with the introduction of Librium® (chlordiazepoxide). Sometimes called "tranquilizers," Valium® is one of the most well-know examples. Like many other psychiatric drugs, these also affect the brain's neurotransmitters, in this case by activating GABA (gamma aminobutyric acid), a neurotransmitter that reduces anxiety. Klonopin® (clonazepam) is the benzodiazepine that has been most studied for use in treating social anxiety. Even though they have shown some effectiveness, these drugs are not usually prescribed for long-term treatment of social anxiety disorder. When they are used, medical practitioners generally limit the time one can be on them because of their addictive qualities and withdrawal symptoms.

The possibility of addiction is especially troubling if the patient is already abusing alcohol or other drugs. Some physicians think the fear of addiction to benzodiazepines has been exaggerated. They believe it is unlikely that most individuals who are prescribed benzodiazepines as treatment for social anxiety disorder and remain under close supervision of the prescribing physician would develop an addiction to these medications.

Other possible side effects include headaches, dizziness, lightheadedness, confusion and forgetfulness, nervousness, unsteadiness, sexual problems, fatigue and drowsiness, or insomnia.

Benzodiazepines are fast-acting medications. Within thirty minutes (sometimes as little as fifteen minutes) of ingesting one of these drugs, a person will generally notice a decrease in anxiety. Therefore, a benzodiazepine is sometimes prescribed to give immediate relieve from symptoms while a patient is waiting for an antidepressant to take effect.

Other Medications

Fast-acting medications called beta-blockers (beta-adrenergic receptor blocking agents) were first introduced in the 1960s

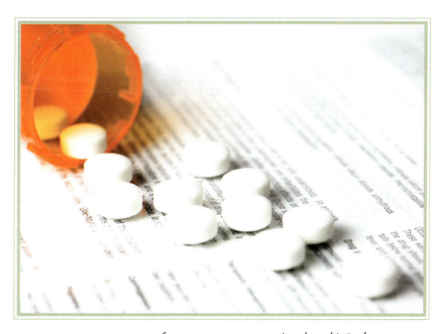

Drug manufacturers are required to list the possible side effects on a packaging insert.

to treat high blood pressure, but today they are sometimes prescribed to counteract bothersome physical symptoms associated with social anxiety. Uncontrollable trembling and rapid
heartbeat are examples of symptoms that could be treated
by these prescription drugs. Inderal® (propanolol) and Te-
normin® (atenolol) are beta-blockers that might be used for

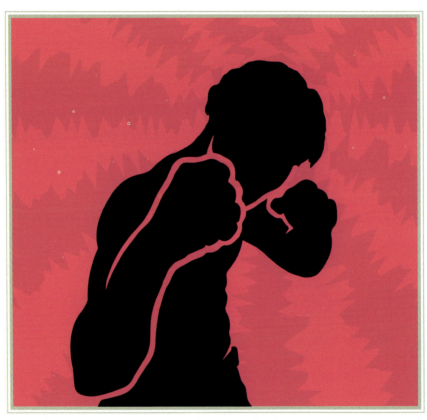

*Adrenaline causes the "fight-or-flight" reaction, getting
the body ready to either face danger or run away; however,
a person with social anxiety will experience the same
"adrenaline rush" from social situations, where in most
cases, the person can neither fight nor run away—but is
left with a pounding heart and accelerated breathing.*

this purpose. Beta-blockers work quickly (within thirty minutes) to "block" specific nerve-cell receptors (known as the "beta" receptors) located on organs and muscles by attaching themselves to those receptors. Essentially, they block the adrenaline, thus inhibiting responses usually caused by this hormone. When they attach themselves to nerve-cell receptors on the heart and sweat glands, for example, they prevent the accelerated heartbeat and profuse sweating dreaded by some people with social anxiety. As with other drugs, doctors must consider all a patient's medical conditions when deciding on treatment. People with asthma, diabetes, or heart disease should not be given beta-blockers. Beta-blockers are not antidepressants. They are most often used as a "temporary fix" for physical symptoms associated with performance anxiety (for example, to control the trembling hands of someone who must give speeches at conferences). They are not effective treatments for the more constant symptoms manifested in social anxiety disorder or for psychological fears associated with it.

A scientific study has also shown an anti-***epilepsy*** medication (not a beta-blocker) called Neurontin® (gabapentin) to be effective for treating social anxiety disorder.

BuSpar® (buspirone) is a drug that generally reduces anxiety within two to four weeks of use, but does not fall into previously discussed categories. Both dopamine and serotonin appear to be affected. It has been prescribed mainly for specific social anxieties and should not be prescribed in combination with MAOIs.

Examples of Drugs That Have Been Used to Treat Social Anxiety

Selective Serotonin Reuptake Inhibitors (SSRIs)

Celexa® (citalopram)

Lexapro® (escitalopram) (available in the United States but not in Canada)

Paxil and Paxil CR® (paroxetine)

Prozac (fluoxetine) (also marketed as Sarafem® and Prozac Weekly®)

Zoloft (sertraline)

Serotonin and Norepinephrine Reuptake Inhibitor (SNRI)

Effexor and Effexor XR® (venlafaxine and venlafaxine hydrochloride)

Cymbalta® (duloxetine)

Monoamine Oxidase Inhibitors (MAOIs)

Marplan® (isocarboxazid)

Nardil® (phenelzine)

Parnate® (tranylcypromine)

TCA (Tricyclic Antidepressant)

Tofranil (imipramine)

Benzodiazepines

Activan® (lorczepam)

Klonopin® (clonazepam) (available as Rivitrol® in Canada)

Lectopam® (bromazepam) (available in Canada but not in the United States)

Serax® (oxazepam)

Valium® (diazepam)

Xanax® and Xanax XR® (alprazolam)

Several treatments are available for social anxiety disorder, but many people delay seeking help. It is easy to understand why someone with this condition would be reluctant to contact a doctor or mental-health professional. Just making the phone call to get an appointment or needing to describe symptoms over the phone could cause escalating anxiety and avoidance behavior. According to Dr. Eric Hollander and Nicholas Bakalar, coauthors of *Coping with Social Anxiety: The Definitive Guide to Effective Treatment Options*:

> On average, a person suffers with social anxiety for fifteen years before seeking any professional intervention, and even then most people go to the doctor not because of their social anxiety, but because they are suffering from comorbid disorders like depression or panic disorder.

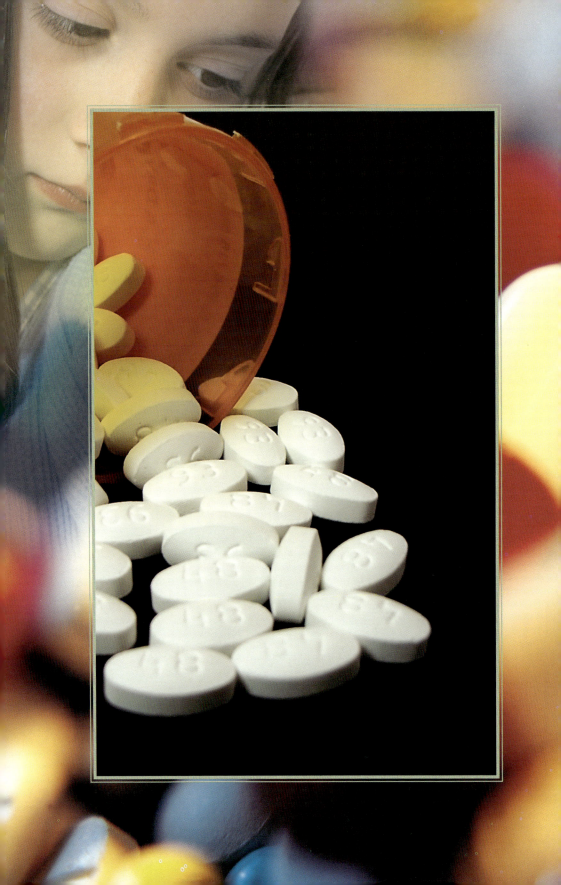

Chapter 4

More About Antidepressants

Dear Scared All the Time,

I can relate to some of the things you describe. I started college last fall, but now I'm home and preparing to start all over again. Here's how I ended up leaving college after only three months.

First of all, I only had a couple of good friends in high school, and I didn't get into the colleges they chose. Let's face it, I only picked those colleges because I was afraid of going away alone.

Next, the college roommate who had been assigned to me moved his stuff into the room, and never came back! I met him when we were moving in—then nothing. I wondered why he was never there and concluded I must have made a really rotten impression. I was counting on getting

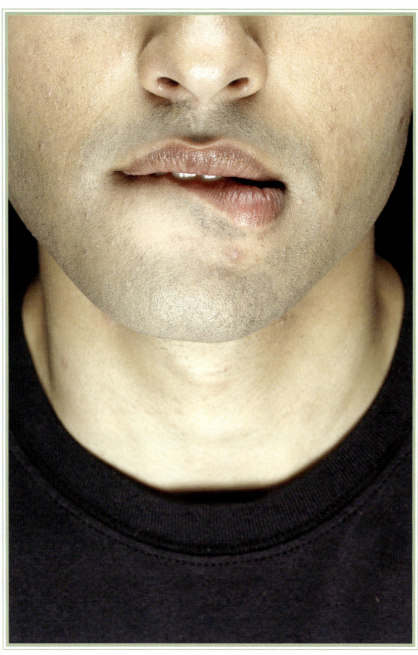

When a person is so self-conscious that he is unable to engage in normal social interactions, he may have a social anxiety disorder.

to know my roommate; I figured he'd be the first friend I'd make at school. I felt really funny about the whole thing. Turns out he lived only thirty miles from the college, and even though he paid for housing on campus, he never used it. Go figure. Unfortunately, I didn't find out about that until I was ready to leave college, but I'm jumping ahead of myself. Back to the story:

To make matters worse, my room was on a floor with mostly older students. They already had friends, and none of them seemed interested in making friends with me. A couple of times I forced myself to go to the lounge to watch TV, and the one or two people who were already there got up and left. Honest. I've always been uncomfortable around people, but at this point I started to feel like I had leprosy or something.

Classes weren't any better, and I had no one to eat with in the cafeteria. I got more and more self-conscious. I couldn't stand the loneliness, but I felt less and less capable of making friends. I called my parents to tell them how lonely I was, and they insisted I see a campus counselor. I forced myself to do that and explained to the counselor that I was getting more and more depressed. After I gave permission, she telephoned my parents and told them I could benefit from an evaluation by a psychiatrist. Then I called my parents and basically begged to go home. I think they were scared I'd commit suicide or something, so they said yes.

Because of our medical insurance plan, my parents had to call our general-care physician to request a referral. Instead of referring me to a psychiatrist, she sent me to another psychologist. He asked questions about how I was feeling, what my concerns were, and how I thought he could help me. I told him I was depressed, and he asked whether I'd felt that way during previous times of my life. I had to admit that I had. He explained treatment options, which included the possibility of taking medication, although psychologists like him can't prescribe them.

I'm getting treatment now, but I'm not going to tell you what it is. Maybe you'll think that's weird, but everybody's different, and what worked for me probably won't work for you. The point is that you need to talk to somebody who really knows about these things—like a psychologist or psychiatrist. I wish I would have done that while I was still in high school. I've been able to get a job, and I'm feeling better now. I'm going to start taking classes at our local community college, and I really think I'm going to be okay. Wish me luck, and I'll wish you the same.

Sincerely,
College Bound

Should Antidepressants Be Used to Treat Social Anxiety?

All of us experience situations that can decrease our self-esteem, increase our social anxieties, and make us feel depressed. Sometimes these feelings lessen over time. As people get older, many are able to place situations in proper

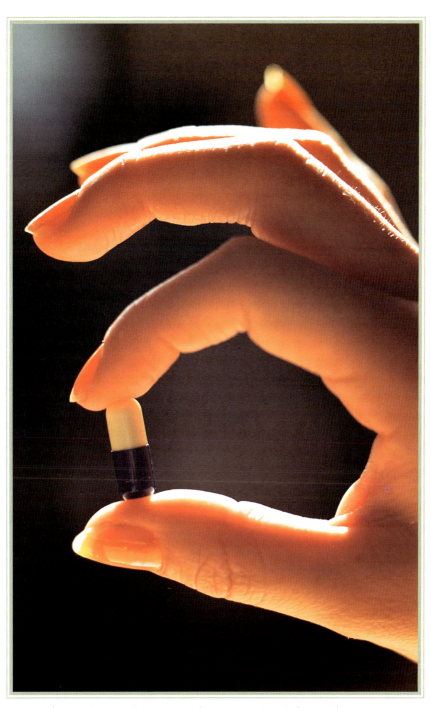

Should social anxiety be treated with medication?

perspective, assigning them an appropriate level of importance or irrelevance in their lives. Other times bad experiences pile up on top of each other, and their cumulative effect can make everything seem worse.

Many people wonder if social anxiety should ever be treated with prescription drugs. The following testimony, given at a hearing conducted by the FDA in 2004, provides a good example of the dangers of prescribing SSRIs for treatment of simple shyness or mild depression:

> The two minutes I have to speak will not permit me to go into the details of what I suffered while taking Prozac, Paxil, and Zoloft from age twelve to eighteen. . . . I went from being a shy and mildly depressed but never suicidal kid, to being overcome with thoughts of hurting and killing myself while on the SSRI drugs, thoughts which I acted on. Since quitting SSRIs over a decade ago, I have never again self-mutilated or had suicidal thoughts. All other things being equal, the suicidality simply vanished. For me, this is clear proof that the drugs must have played a role, and I am one of the lucky ones; I have lived to tell the tale.

The person providing this testimony describes herself as having been a shy kid with mild depression, and she blames SSRIs for making her worse. The situation is not clearly black and white, however, with SSRIs always being a bad idea for people with social anxiety. In its most serious form, social anxiety disorder can lead to avoidance behaviors, drug abuse, or serious depression, even suicide. In her book *Diagonally-Parked in a Parallel Universe: Working Through Social Anxiety,* social psychologist Signe A. Dayhoff reports that from 40 percent to 50 percent of those seeking treatment for social anxiety disorder also have major depression. In cases where patients are already at high risk for suicide, many medical professionals consider medication essential.

Right or wrong, antidepressants are the most frequently prescribed drugs for treatment of social anxiety disorder. They usually work more quickly than other therapies, and they may offer at least temporary relief for individuals who are so distraught they are contemplating ending their life.

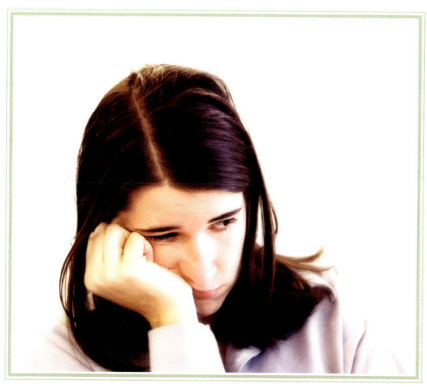

From 40 to 50 percent of all people seeking treatment for social anxiety disorder are also clinically depressed.

But antidepressants are also associated with risks, including the possibility of increased depression and suicidal thoughts. Therefore, it is very important that medical practitioners and patients carefully weigh all potential risks against actual needs. When antidepressants are prescribed, the medical practitioner and parents or other caregivers must closely monitor the patient for any signs of adverse reactions.

Why Antidepressants Work—Or Do They?

If either an excess or a deficiency of certain neurotransmitters causes a mental disorder, antidepressants may work to correct this chemical imbalance, thus diminishing problem feelings and symptoms. Sometimes the temporary use of antide-

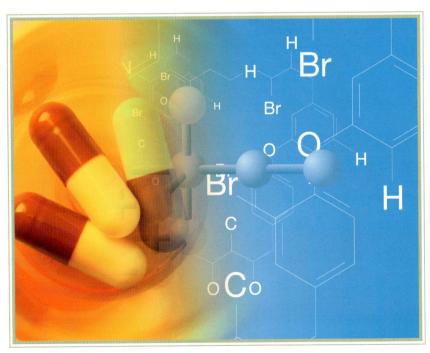

Antidepressants are chemicals that affect brain chemistry.

pressants or other medications can lessen anxiety symptoms enough to allow people to modify their avoidance behaviors. If a person feels capable of attending a conference, for example, and then experiences a positive outcome from performing that task, he may feel less anxious the next time a similar situation is encountered.

Antidepressants can be dangerous, however, and they do not have the same level of effectiveness for everyone. In fact, many **clinical trials** of these medications have not proven their effectiveness. Yet they do seem to help many people. However, determining which medication and what dosage will work for a specific individual, if it will even help at all, can take a considerable amount of time. A person's tolerance level for different antidepressants also varies. Consequently,

Who Can Prescribe Psychiatric Drugs?

• *physicians who have an M.D.*

• *psychiatrists (These professionals have obtained an M.D.)*

• *some health-care professionals who work under the direction of a medical doctor, such as psychiatric nurse practitioners*

• *in New Mexico only: psychologists who have obtained specific additional training*

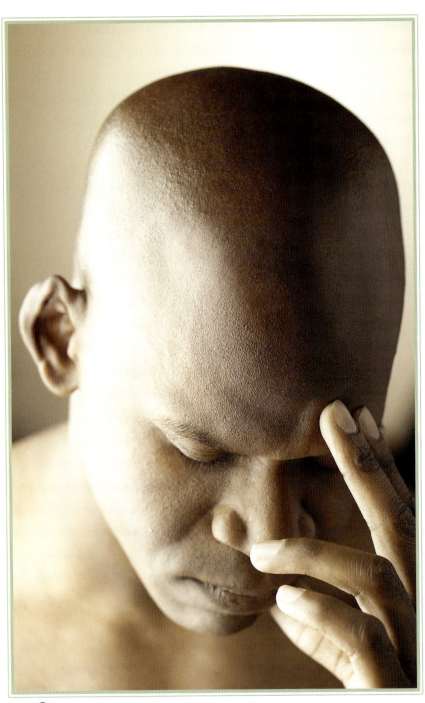

Headache is just one of the side effects that SSRIs can cause.

when these drugs are prescribed, they are usually prescribed at a low dose, and then the dosage is increased over time until the **optimum** level is achieved.

Risks and Side Effects

The possibility of negative side effects exists with most prescription medications including antidepressants. Many people can take antidepressants without experiencing any adverse effects, but other people will notice one or more.

SSRIs

Side effects vary with the different SSRIs, but in general, a person taking one could notice any of the following: dizziness, headaches, nausea, sweating, increased agitation and jitteriness, or she might become fatigued and drowsy. Some people may notice dry mouth or increased thirst, experience chest pain or heart palpitations, or gain weight as side effects of these medications.

Taking a look at the two SSRIs that have obtained official FDA approval for treatment of social phobia, we see that possible side effects for Paxil include dizziness, nervousness, yawning, drowsiness, insomnia, dry mouth, reduced appetite, nausea, constipation or diarrhea, sweating, tremors, infections, and sexual problems. According to RxList, the Internet Drug Index, Paxil can also have more serious side effects, including impulsivity, panic attacks, **hypomania**, and **mania**. Paxil CR is reported to have fewer side effects than the other form of Paxil, since it is absorbed by the small intestine rather than the stomach. Zoloft can cause dry mouth, nausea, and

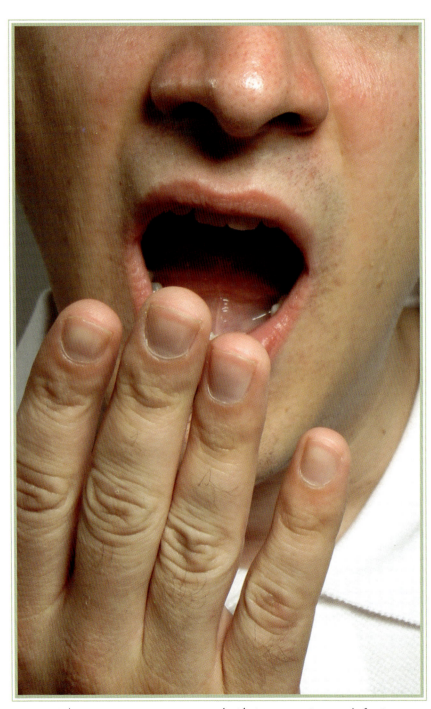

Antidepressants may cause both insomnia and fatigue.

insomnia. Additionally, a person taking it might experience diarrhea or sexual problems.

Effexor XR (an SNRI) can have side effects similar to those caused by SSRIs, including dry mouth, loss of appetite, constipation, insomnia, weakness, and sexual problems.

MAOIs

An individual taking an MAOI might experience some of the same side effects as a person taking another type of antidepressant, including dry mouth, headache, dizziness, weakness, drowsiness and fatigue, insomnia, jitteriness, weight

Black-Box Warnings

Two dozen studies involving more than four thousand children and adolescents now suggest that some children who are treated with antidepressants can experience increased suicidal thoughts and behaviors. Nine different antidepressants were involved in these studies. None of the subjects in the studies committed suicide during the time of the trials, but the risk of having suicidal thoughts or possible behaviors was 4 percent as compared with a 2 percent risk for subjects who were given placebos.

The FDA now requires all antidepressants to carry a black-box warning stating that children and adolescents taking these drugs may have an increased risk of suicide. Black-box warnings are printed in a black frame on package inserts and promotional materials. They indicate the FDA has determined the product has the highest risk among prescription medications.

gain, constipation, and sexual problems. Potentially lethal side effects are possible if the user ingests certain other medicines or even some foods while taking an MAOI. The possibility of headaches, vomiting, and a serious rise in blood pressure, even a stroke, are possible when these medications are combined with wine, beer, and foods containing *tyramine*. Some of these foods include yogurt, aged cheese, overripe bananas, figs, raisins, avocados, chocolate, soy sauce, tofu, sauerkraut, some beans, and some fish and meat. This remains a concern up to two weeks after discontinuing use of the medication.

TCAs

Side effects of TCAs can include dry mouth, constipation, blurred vision, and drowsiness.

In general, side effects of antidepressant use may be entirely absent or they can range from simply annoying to serious. People taking antidepressants should avoid alcohol, take doses of their medication as prescribed, and avoid specific foods if directed to do so. If side effects develop, the individual's physician needs to be notified immediately. All side effects should be discussed with the prescribing physician before beginning and while taking any medication. Having some side effects does not necessarily mean the patient will have to discontinue use of the drug, as the side effects might be tolerated, diminish with continued use, or be managed with use of other medications. Sometimes, however, side effects do prevent a patient from continuing on a particular medication, even if it is helping to reduce anxiety symptoms.

Coming Off Antidepressants

A person who is taking an antidepressant for social anxiety disorder will typically do so for six to twelve months. Sometimes treatment with antidepressants will last longer. When use is discontinued, it is done so gradually. This reduces the possibility and severity of withdrawal symptoms. The more

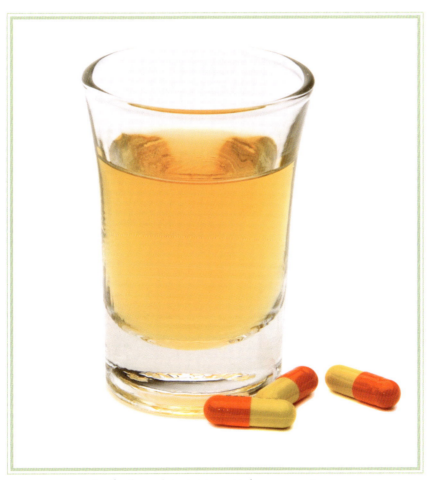

Alcohol and MAOI antidepressants can be a dangerous combination.

quickly an SSRI is **metabolized** by the body, the more likely it is to cause withdrawal symptoms with discontinued use. For example, because Paxil is metabolized quickly, withdrawal symptoms could be more noticeable than some of the other SSRIs. Withdrawal symptoms for Paxil could include mood fluctuations, nausea, sweating, dizziness, headache, fatigue or nervousness and agitation, abnormal dreams and sleep disturbances, ringing or buzzing in the ears, even electric shock sensations. Prozac stays in the system longer than other SSRIs; this feature can decrease the likelihood of withdrawal symptoms. Nevertheless, one could experience sweating, agitation, jitteriness, dry mouth, nausea, vomiting, insomnia, diarrhea, and sexual problems. Someone withdrawing too quickly from a serotonin antagonist might experience flu-like symptoms.

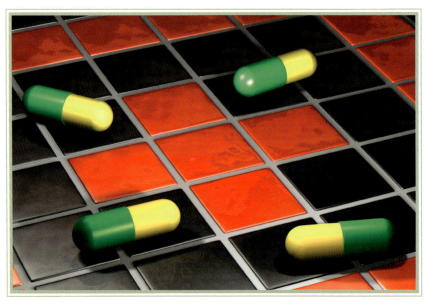

Medication should not be viewed as a permanent cure for social anxiety disorder.

Regardless of the particular drug being discontinued, the patient should report any negative symptoms to the prescribing physician so they can be properly managed.

Antidepressants and other medications should not be thought of as a "cure" for social anxiety disorder. While they may lessen one's anxiety, it could return when the medication is discontinued. Those with social anxiety disorder who elect to take prescription medications as part of their treatment are most likely to experience lasting improvement when medication is combined with therapies aimed at behavioral modification, such as cognitive-behavioral therapy.

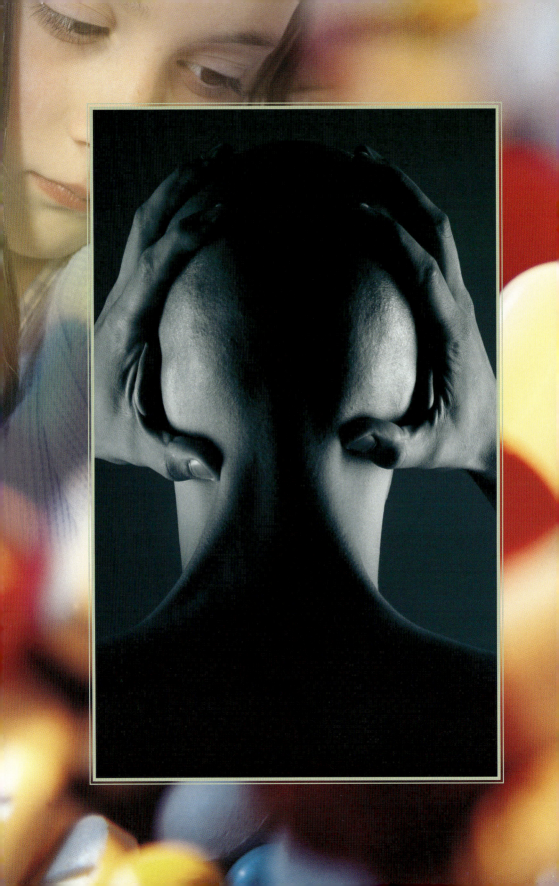

Chapter 5

More About Cognitive-Behavioral Therapy

Dear Scared All the Time,

I've been wondering how much I'm like you. I don't avoid parties, in fact I enjoy them, and I love to shop, but there are a couple things kind of strange about me. I don't think they're serious, but I wonder why I'm like this, and I sure hope I don't get any worse. The thing is, I can't bring myself to use my cell phone if anyone is anywhere near me. In fact, I can't use any telephone unless I'm alone. Don't laugh. It seems like a small thing, but it's pretty weird. I can't call my mother at the appointed time when I'm at the mall unless I leave the store ahead of time and find a secluded place somewhere. It's a real hassle, and when I'm with friends, it's embarrassing. I've tried to cure myself of this craziness, but it seems impossible. And please don't say I need professional help. The thing there is that I hate talking to higher-ups, you know, people that are "superiors." They make me really jittery. I get all stressed out and then I can't talk straight. Do you think there's a pill or something I can take for this?

—Reluctant Phone Gal

Understanding Yourself

Reluctant Phone Gal understands she has a problem, but it does not sound serious enough to warrant medication. When someone engages in avoidant behavior (for example, not attending social gatherings, missing work, not talking on the phone in public places), the anxiety they'll experience at having to participate in those activities in the future is likely to increase. People can get into a sort of "circle of avoidance," where having avoided one situation reinforces their desire to avoid the next similar one. The best course of action is to seek the therapy needed to face social fears. This can be a healthy first step toward getting social anxiety under permanent control.

First developed in the 1960s, cognitive-behavioral therapy provides a **systematic** method of **progressive** steps to assist in this goal, and it is safe to use in treating any minor unwanted shyness, specific social phobias, and generalized social anxiety disorder. Since each person is unique, cognitive-behavioral therapy should be tailored to meet individual requirements. Most people with social anxiety disorder can expect to need from twelve to twenty sessions, with practice and assignments (homework) performed between them. Several weeks of treatment might be necessary before the client begins to notice significant change.

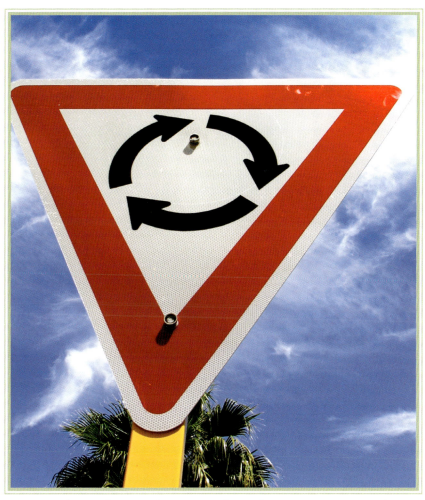

People with social anxiety disorder can get trapped in a "circle of avoidance," where each feared situation leads to greater fear of the next similar situation.

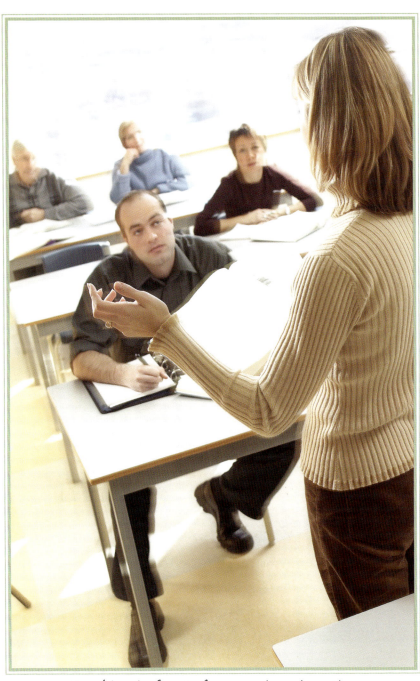

*Speaking in front of a group is a situation
that makes many people feel anxious.*

First Steps at the Therapist's Office

The therapist will ask the client a series of questions to determine a **hierarchy** of situations that cause anxiety. For example, the patient may be only mildly anxious while shopping but extremely nervous if she has to return an item to the store. The therapist will want to know about the physical symptoms she experiences while anticipating as well as while engaging in the various stress-causing situations.

The patient may be asked to keep a diary where she lists all her anxiety-causing situations as they occur and the degree of discomfort associated with them. For example, she might be extremely anxious at the thought of introducing herself at a party and even experience chest pain while walking into the event but only feel mildly anxious while sitting alone and observing the gathering. Or a person who is so worried about reading aloud in class that she begins to fumble over the words might be only mildly concerned about answering a question in front of classmates. Maybe the thought of being asked to give her opinion makes her throat feel like it's constricting, and she fears her mind will go blank. Perhaps she is so scared that she skips school when she is expected to present her opinions.

When the therapist and client understand exactly which experiences cause anxiety and the degree of anxiety experienced, they can decide on a chronology for treatment—which things they want to work on first, second, and so on. This will be determined by several factors, including which situations are most important to the patient and whether some of

Who Can Provide Cognitive-Behavioral Therapy?

• *psychiatrists*

• *psychiatric nurse practitioners*

• *social workers*

• *psychologists*

• *other mental-health counselors*

them can be conquered easily. Experiencing success at conquering easier situations can build the patient's confidence to overcome increasingly difficult ones. On the other hand, some items may occur so rarely in the person's life that they can be removed from the list entirely.

Examples of "Distorted Thinking"

People with social anxiety disorder commonly overexaggerate the likelihood something will go wrong in a given situation. Here's an example: Robert has extreme anxiety each time he has to take a test. He fears failure and worries that everyone in class will think he's stupid. Yet the reality is that he has never received a test grade lower than B. Robert is overestimating his likelihood of failure. Furthermore, Robert is making a negative assumption about other people's thoughts. He jumps to

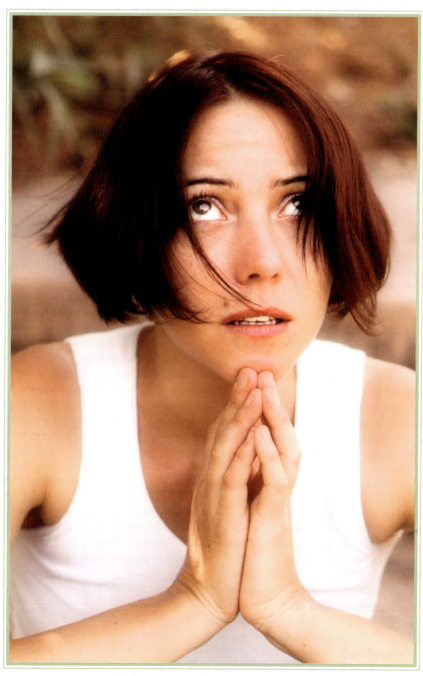

*Cognitive-behavioral therapy helps individuals
break distorted thought habits.*

the conclusion that all his classmates will think poorly of him if he gets a bad grade. In reality, nobody knows the thoughts that are in other people's heads, and it is unlikely that every single classmate will have the same thought.

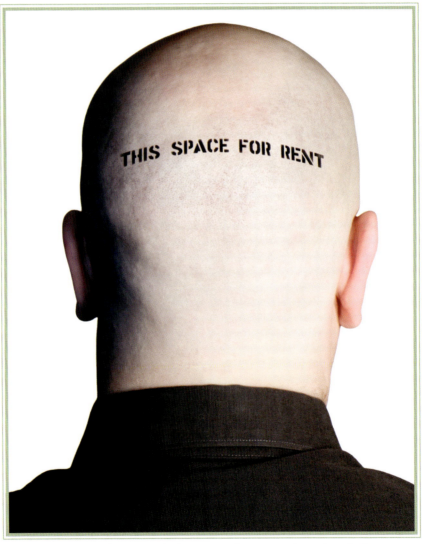

Cognitive-behavioral therapy shows individuals how to choose the thoughts they allow to occupy their minds.

People with social anxiety disorder commonly have per-fectionist tendencies and unreasonable expectations of themselves. They may think it a "weakness" to show any anxiety or nervousness in front of others no matter what the situation is. They often believe that if the humiliation or embarrassment they fear were to happen, it would have catastrophic results. They overestimate the importance of many social situations, the kinds of things that might "go wrong," and people's reactions.

Thoughts and Habits

One of the basic aims of cognitive-behavioral therapy is to replace incorrect and negative thoughts with realistic and positive ones. Usually the anxiety and fear experienced in social anxiety disorder are being caused by an incorrect and exaggerated belief about a situation. Something is being wrongfully interpreted as threatening, hurtful, or dangerous, and this is causing anxiety.

To change these beliefs, patients are asked to determine exactly what their thoughts are concerning anxiety-provoking situations. By discovering "why" particular social occasions are causing anxiety, they learn what it is that they actually fear in each situation. Here's another example: Kayla has anxiety about walking into a party and worries she will trip coming through the door. What is it she actually fears—falling down, being seen falling down, or being judged because she fell down? What does she believe people will think of her if she does fall down—that she's clumsy, that she looks ridiculous, that there's something physically wrong with her, that they would never want to get to know someone that clumsy and ridiculous? Kayla can benefit from considering whether or not her thoughts are realistic. Are these the thoughts she would have if she saw someone fall down at a party, or is it more likely she would be concerned about that person? If she did fall down, what would really happen? Maybe someone would laugh. What would that really mean? How would she feel about that? Is what one person thinks truly important? When was the last time Kayla fell down when entering a room?

Both memory and imagination are useful for determining why various situations cause anxiety. Role playing can be another helpful tool, both in determining anxiety-causing situations and in practicing new reactions to them. Being able to witness role playing or to participate in it is one of the advantages of participation in a cognitive-behavioral therapy group.

Individual or Group

Being in a group is often a part of cognitive-behavioral therapy. Other advantages include meeting people with similar situations. It can help to know you're not the only one going through this, and members of the group can share personal experiences and provide valuable feedback.

Attending a group can be difficult for a person with social anxiety disorder, and it may not be part of everyone's initial treatment. Understanding and working through anxiety as-

Practice Rational Thinking

When you feel anxious about a social situation, ask yourself these questions:

- *What do I fear will happen?*

- *Have I had similar anxious thoughts in the past?*

- *Did the fearful thoughts become reality?*

- *Is the feared event very likely to happen now?*

- *Can I think of other ways to interpret this situation?*

- *How would someone else feel if they were in this position?*

sociated with group attendance can be a goal that a patient works toward.

Changed Thinking

Remember, one goal of cognitive-behavioral therapy is to change negative thoughts to more rational, positive ones. Here's an example: Tom worked hard on his class presentation, but he's extremely nervous about the upcoming event. *I'll lose my place, my mind will go blank, my hands will shake, I'll be totally mortified. Everyone will think I'm a real loser*, he fears. Tom wants to be rid of his negative thoughts and the anxiety they're causing. To do that, he begins to think rationally about the situation: *I know I did enough research about the topic and chose the most interesting information for the report. I practiced presenting the report first in front of a mirror and then in front of my family, and they told me it sounded good. The teacher is allowing us to use our notes during the presentations. If I do lose my place or if my mind goes blank, I can look through my notes. If my hands shake, no one will see them because I'll be using a podium and my hands will be hidden by that. I've noticed other people's hands shake sometimes, and I didn't give it a second thought. It is unlikely "everything" will go wrong. It is unlikely that I'll be "totally mortified" by my performance. If I do make a mistake "everyone" in class will not think I'm a "loser." Most people in class will probably like the report. Others will be so worried about giving their own reports that they might not pay much attention to mine. What do I really care if someone in class doesn't like my report? That person might not be interested in the topic. That wouldn't mean he has any negative personal feelings about me.*

Positive Thoughts to Keep Things in Perspective

• *No one is perfect.*

• *It's okay if everyone doesn't like me.*

• *Anxiety symptoms are uncomfortable, but they're not dangerous.*

• *People aren't noticing most of the stuff I'm worrying about.*

• *This situation isn't that important; six months from now, it will only be a distant memory.*

If negative thoughts continue to interfere with his thinking, Tom could use another tactic: He could tell himself to "stop thinking about those things right now" and schedule a time to think about them later.

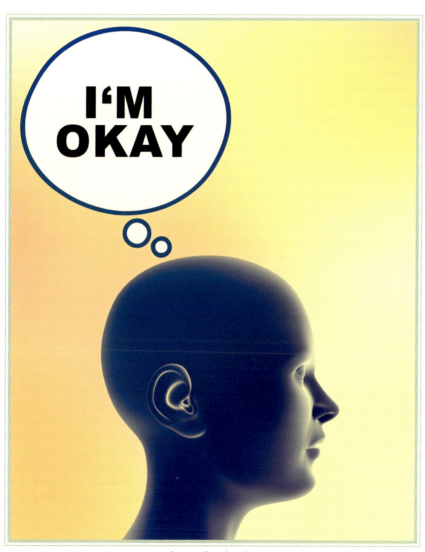

Positive thought habits can help individuals conquer social anxiety.

Exposure to Social Situations

Remember this is cognitive-*behavioral* therapy. The goal is to modify both thoughts and behaviors. Deliberately exposing yourself to feared social situations in order to change your beliefs and behaviors may be very difficult. This can be approached by gradual exposure the person can handle, but there's no avoiding this part of the therapy. To prepare, the patient will spend time visualizing a social situation and working through it successfully in her imagination before tackling it for real. The therapist will be involved in selection, preparation, and approach to be certain the client experiences a successful outcome. Exposing oneself to feared social situations until anxiety subsides is essential to long-term success. After facing a social situation successfully, it can be helpful to record details about it for future reference. Client and therapist will undoubtedly discuss the event, and together they'll decide when to repeat the exposure and when to move on to another social situation. Repeat exposure is necessary to continue reducing anxiety and to maintain success in keeping it under control.

Managing Thoughts and Behaviors

Successful completion of cognitive-behavioral therapy is no guarantee the patient will never again experience social anxiety. But when anxious feelings do appear, the person will be better prepared to realistically evaluate his feelings, replace negative thoughts with positive ones, and resist any temptation to fall into avoidant behaviors.

Examples of Other Treatments and Technologies

Social Skills Training: With this training, people learn about facial expressions, tone of voice, gestures, proper posture, making eye contact, and other aspects of communicating effectively with others. Improving these skills can boost confidence and make social interactions more successful.

Virtual Technology: Therapists began using this technology in the 1990s. Today it is used to treat numerous mental disorders, including anxiety caused by public speaking. Virtual technology can be beneficial for imagination and role-playing aspects of therapy.

While cognitive-behavioral therapy is usually very effective in treating social anxiety disorder, it might not work for everyone. People spend years developing their thought patterns, and it can take a considerable amount of time and work to change them. There may be occasional setbacks as one progresses toward recovery. Rather than becoming discouraged when this happens, it's important to remember minor setbacks are to be expected and to continue working with the therapist. Therapists can employ many techniques to meet individual needs. In the meantime, there are things we can all do to reduce our levels of stress.

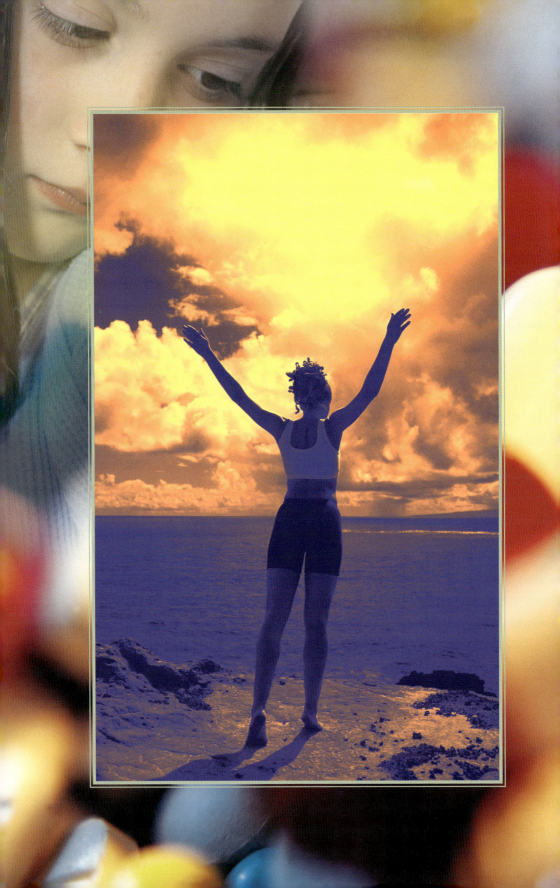

Chapter 6

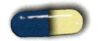

More Ways to Help Yourself and Some Things to Avoid

Wow! Thanks to everyone who responded to my posting.

I feel bad for what so many of you are going through, but it really has helped to discover I'm not the only one. I've started reading a book about social anxiety disorder, and for the first time, I feel like I can beat this thing. I've taken the advice some of you gave me and made an appointment to speak with a psychologist in two weeks. I'm encouraged about my prospects. I also decided now is a good time to get other parts of my life in order. You know the "eat right and exercise for all-around health" kind of stuff. Who knows, maybe that's part of the reason I'm having a better outlook on everything. Anyway, it can't hurt, right? I'll write again after I see the psychologist. In the meantime, thanks again for your help.

—No Longer Scared All the Time

Can Eating Right and Exercise Help?

Long-term, consistent exposure to stress and anxiety can increase a person's susceptibility to illnesses such as heart disease. For those with social anxiety disorder, conquering anxiety-inducing behaviors through cognitive-behavioral therapy has proven successful. There is no evidence that simply eating a healthy diet or developing good exercise habits will reduce social anxiety, but everyone can improve their overall physical and mental health by doing these things, which may help reduce stress.

Food Allergies

Surprising as it may seem, allergies to some foods can affect a person's mood. Irritability, anxiety, and depression are only some of the symptoms an individual could experience when eating a food to which she is allergic. Chocolate, citrus fruits, wheat, dairy products, eggs, soy products, and peanuts are common allergy sources. If you suspect you have a food allergy, you can test it out by avoiding the food to see how that makes you feel, but it's best to discuss it with your doctor.

Diet

Caffeine is a stimulant, and beverages and foods containing it can impact one's mood. Most people are able to drink one or two cups of coffee or green or black tea without negative consequences, and these beverages can even have some health benefits. However, those who notice increased agitation and anxiety when using these substances may want to moderate

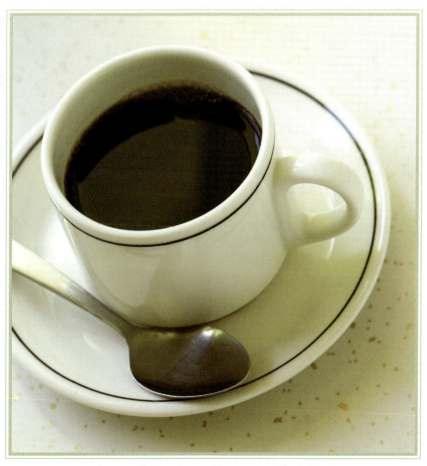

The caffeine in coffee can affect brain chemicals, increasing social anxiety.

or discontinue their use. Caffeine can affect norepinephrine levels and decrease the amount of calcium and B vitamins available in the body. These vitamins play an important role in the health of the central nervous system.

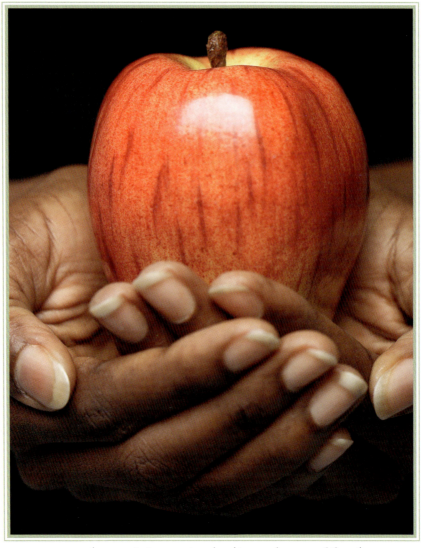

Good nutrition—including plenty of fresh fruits—can help the brain function optimally.

Food for Thought

Do Americans today live in a society that devalues shyness?
Do we reward aggressive behaviors over shy ones?
Do video games and movies reflect an admiration for aggressive behaviors?
Does widespread use of the Internet for communicating with friends (even local friends) through e-mail and instant messenger, and use of cell phones for text messaging, discourage face-to-face and voice-to-voice social contacts, thus encouraging social anxieties?

Eating healthful foods promotes good health. To obtain vitamin B_1 (thiamine), eat whole-wheat products, peanuts, peas, beans, fish, and meat. For B_2 (riboflavin), eat leafy green vegetables, dairy products, eggs, and meat. For B_3 (niacin), eat whole grains, peanuts, fish, and meat. For B_6 (pyridoxine), eat bran products, bananas, potatoes, lentils, turkey, and liver. The B vitamin choline is found in oatmeal, wheat germ, egg yolk, cabbage, cauliflower, soybeans, and liver. The B vitamins are most helpful when obtained together.

Sugar can also negatively impact the body's levels of B vitamins and can have other powerful effects on the body because of the way it affects ***insulin*** levels. Remember that the brain's neurotransmitters are derived from amino acids. Insulin affects amino acids in the following way: Serotonin is derived from an amino acid called tryptophan. Insulin causes amino acids, with the exception of tryptophan, to be absorbed by the body's muscles and tissues. This, in turn, results in more tryptophan, which is converted to serotonin, being available to the brain compared to other neurotransmitters. This can produce a calming effect, and it may be why so many of us turn to sugar in times of stress. Sometimes people eat too much refined sugar, however, and experience unpleasant physical symptoms as a result of a spike in insulin levels. These symptoms can include agitation, irritability, and an increased heart rate.

It is important to include foods containing vitamin C (readily available in citrus fruits), calcium (good sources include dairy products, leafy green vegetables, salmon, and sardines), and amino acids (available in many foods including dairy products, beans, root vegetables, sunflower seeds, meat, and fish) in one's diet, as a lack of these nutrients may result in increased stress.

Using Herbs

Unless you consult with a medical doctor and obtain her agreement to supervise herbal treatment, it is best to avoid trying to treat anxiety and depression with these substances. Although the word "herb" sounds harmless because we use culinary herbs when cooking, some of these plants have powerful drug-like qualities. They may be troublesome when used alone and dangerous when combined with other medications, especially SSRIs, MAOIs, and the other prescription treatments used for social anxiety disorder. Examples of herbs to be wary of include the following.

St. John's Wort

Pretty yellow flowers and delicate leaves that look like they're sprinkled with pepper belie the power behind St. John's wort. Like antidepressant drugs, this plant is thought to alter the amount of serotonin available to the brain. In many countries, the herb is used as a treatment for anxiety and depression, and studies have shown that it can be an effective treatment

Herbal Remedies

Here are a few things to be aware of when considering use of herbal remedies:

- *Herbs are not regulated by the federal government.*

- *There is no assurance that herbal strengths listed on product labels are accurate.*

- *Anyone can purchase herbs without a prescription.*

- *The effectiveness of most herbal remedies in treating specific conditions has not been widely tested.*

- *How various herbs react with prescription medications is not well understood.*

- *The safety of using most herbs is not known.*

for some people. Possible side effects include dry mouth, dizziness, rashes, itching, sensitivity to light, digestive problems, and restlessness or fatigue.

Kava Kava

Studies have indicated that the root of this variety of pepper plant may reduce both anxiety and depression in some people. Kava dermopathy is the name of a rash that can develop as a side effect at some dosage levels. The possibility of increased cholesterol and a rise in liver enzymes are other concerns, as is the possibility of a decrease in blood serum and plasma protein.

Exercise

Some people reduce anxiety by practicing yoga or various forms of meditation. Others do it through vigorous exercise. When we feel stressed, our muscles become tense. Regular exercise relieves muscle tension, but the benefits go way beyond that. Maybe you've heard runners talking about running through the pain, until their "endorphins kick in." These hormones are located in the brain where they decrease feelings of pain and increase one's sense of well-being. Besides increasing your endorphins, exercise can increase norepinephrine and help the body metabolize adrenaline. Even that's not all, however. Regular exercise has many more health benefits, including possibly decreasing weight, cholesterol, and blood pressure, while increasing one's memory and ability to concentrate.

Avoiding Drug and Alcohol Abuse

Many people with social anxiety disorder try to self-medicate; in other words, they try to treat their symptoms with alcohol, marijuana, or some other drug. These addictive chemicals may temporarily numb the feelings of anxiety, but in the long run, they make the disorder worse by producing depression and generalized anxiety, which in term can cause still more social avoidant behaviors.

Breathing Right

Perhaps you've noticed a change in your breathing pattern during times of stress. We tend to take smaller, shallow breaths

The Mysterious Blush

In their book The Hidden Face of Shyness: Understanding & Overcoming Social Anxiety, *authors Franklin Schneier, M.D., and Lawrence Welkowitz, Ph.D., point out what an intriguing phenomenon blushing is. Adrenalin plays a role in this occurrence, but it is different from the fight-or-flight response described in chapter 1. In the presence of danger, the walls of blood vessels located just beneath the skin on some parts of the body often constrict, resulting in a pale look rather than a red one. Blushing happens when these same vessels relax and fill with more blood than usual. According to Schneier and Welkowitz, because of this difference, blushing may hold a key to understanding the mechanisms behind social fear as opposed to real physical danger.*

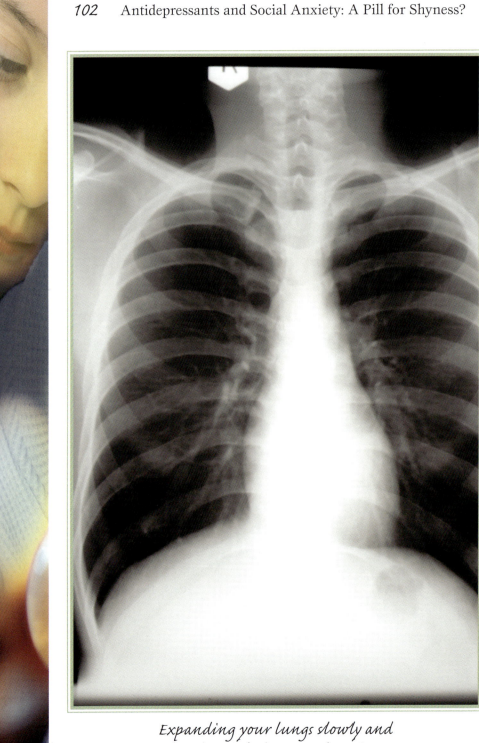

*Expanding your lungs slowly and
deeply can help control anxiety.*

when feeling anxious. You may be able to calm yourself at times like this by taking a few deep breaths. Do this in the following way: As you slowly take in air, send it down into your abdomen. You will see your abdomen swell first, followed by your chest. Hold the breath for a second or two before slowly exhaling. That's all there is to it. It's healthful to do this a few times every day, even when you're not feeling stressed.

The definition of social anxiety disorder has been evolving for over twenty-five years since social phobia was first included in the DSM in 1980. Yet some people still question its validity or don't take it seriously. They believe people with the disorder should just "get over it," "pull themselves together," and "stop acting ridiculous." They fear we may be using drugs and other treatments to "alter people's personalities." Most people who have undergone successful treatment for social anxiety disorder do not feel their personality has been altered; instead, they believe they are finally able to let their personality out. Many of them felt trapped by a debilitating shyness that kept them separated from the world. With each passing year, more people understand the difference between shyness and the severest form of social anxiety disorder. Hopefully, one day soon everyone who is suffering with this condition will seek treatment, thus taking the first steps toward permanent improvement of their lives.

Further Reading

Antony, Martin M., and Richard P. Swinson. *The Shyness & Social Anxiety Workbook: Proven Techniques for Overcoming Your Fears.* Oakland, Calif.: New Harbinger Publications, Inc., 2000.

Appleton, William S. *The New Antidepressants and Antianxieties: What You Need to Know about Zoloft, Paxil, Wellbutrin, Effexor, Clonazepam, Ambien, and More.* New York: Plume, 2004.

Blyth, Jamie, and Jenna Glatzer. *Fear Is No Longer My Reality: How I Overcame Panic and Social Anxiety Disorder—and You Can Too.* New York: McGraw-Hill, 2005.

Breggin, Peter R. *The Anti-Depressant Fact Book: What Your Doctor Won't Tell You about Prozac, Zoloft, Paxil, Celexa and Luvox.* Cambridge, Mass.: Da Capo Press, 2001.

Dayhoff, Signe A. *Diagonally-Parked in a Parallel Universe: Working Through Social Anxiety.* Placitas, N.M.: Effectiveness-Plus Publications, 2000.

Hilliard, Erika B. *Living Fully with Shyness and Social Anxiety: A Comprehensive Guide to Gaining Social Confidence.* New York: Marlowe & Company, 2005.

Hollander, Eric, and Nicholas Bakalar. *Coping with Social Anxiety: The Definitive Guide to Effective Treatment Options.* New York: Henry Holt and Company, 2005.

Markway, Barbara C., and Gregory P. Markway. *Painfully Shy: How to Overcome Social Anxiety and Reclaim Your Life.* New York: St. Martins Press, 2001.

Moehn, Heather. *Coping with Social Anxiety.* New York: Rosen, 2001.

Soifer, Steven, George D. Zgourides, Joseph Himle, and Nancy I. Pickering. *Shy Bladder Syndrome: Your Step-by-Step Guide to Overcoming Paruresis.* Oakland, Calif.: New Harbinger Publications, 2001.

For More Information

Anxiety Disorders Association of America
www.adaa.org

The Anxiety Network International Social Anxiety
Homepage
www.anxietynetwork.com/sphome.html

For many facts about social anxiety:
www.socialanxietyfactsforhealth.org

National Association of Cognitive-Behavioral Therapy
For a description of cognitive-behavioral therapy:
www.nacbt.org/whatiscbt.htm
To search for a cognitive-behavioral therapist in your area:
www.nacbt.org/searchfortherapists.asp

Social Anxiety Network
www.social-anxiety-network.com

Social Anxiety Support
www.socialanxietysupport.com

Social Phobia/Social Anxiety Association
www.socialphobia.org

To read about personal experiences with social anxiety:
www.socialanxietyinstitute.org/experiences.htm

Publisher's note:
The Web sites listed on these pages were active at the time of publication.
The publisher is not responsible for Web sites that have changed their
addresses or discontinued operation since the date of publication. The
publisher will review and update the Web-site list upon each reprint.

Glossary

clinical trials: Medical trials to test the effectiveness of a drug by comparing results from those being given the medication to results from similar patients being given a placebo (sugar pill, fake medication).

cognitive: Having to do with mental processes including awareness, perception, interpretation, reasoning, judgment, and memory.

enzyme: A protein that promotes a specific biochemical reaction.

epilepsy: A medical disorder involving episodes of abnormal electrical discharge in the brain and characterized by periodic loss of consciousness and seizures.

exacerbate: Make something worse; increase its severity.

generic: General; descriptive of an entire class or group.

hierarchy: An order of importance within a group.

hypomania: A mild form of mania.

insulin: A hormone used by the body to break down carbohydrates (sugars and starches) and fats.

intervention: To interfere with something so as to alter or hinder an action.

introspective: Tending to make a detailed examination of one's own feelings, thoughts, and motives.

introverted: Tending to be shy and quiet or ill at ease in a group.

mania: Excessive, exaggerated, and crazed sort of gaiety, enthusiasm, and physical activity, even violent, abnormal behavior.

metabolized: Undergone the processes necessary for the body to obtain energy and nutrients to sustain life.

optimum: The point at which something is the most favorable.

perceptions: Neurological processes by which we recognize and interpret information gained through the senses.

peripheral: The outer edges of something, such as the surface of an organ in the body.

progressive: Increasing in extent or severity as it goes along.

psychoanalysis: A psychology treatment method based on the ideas that mental life functions on both the conscious and unconscious levels and that childhood events have a powerful psychological influence throughout life.

selective mutism: Not speaking by choice rather than for some physical reason.

sensory perception: Recognition or interpretation of something through use of the senses.

systematic: Carried out in a methodical and organized manner.

tyramine: A specific amino acid, $C_8H_{11}NO$, an organic compound derived from ammonia.

Bibliography

American Psychiatric Association. *Diagnostic and Statistical Manual of Mental Disorders, Fourth Edition, Text Revision*. Arlington, Va.: American Psychiatric Publishing, Inc., 2004.

Department of Health and Human Services. Food and Drug Administration. Center for Drug Evaluation and Research. Psychopharmacologic Drugs Advisory Committee with the Pediatric Subcommittee of the Anti-Infective Drugs Advisory Committee. http://www.fda.gov/ohrms/dockets/ac/04/transcripts/4006T1.htm.

Effexor. http://www.effexorxr.com.rk: Marlowe & Company, 2005.

Madison Institute of Medicine. http://www.socialanxietyfactsforhealth.org.

Marohn, Stephanie. *The Natural Medicine Guide to Anxiety*. Charlottesville, Va.: Hampton Roads Publishing Company, Inc., 2003.

National Association of Cognitive-Behavioral Therapists. http://www.nacbt.org.

Paxil. http://www.paxil.com.

PsychNet-UK. http://www.psychnet-uk.com/phobia_list/phobialist.html.

RxList. The Internet Drug Index. http://www.rxlist.com/cgi/generic/parox.htm.

Schneier, Franklin, and Lawrence Welkowitz. *The Hidden Face of Shyness: Understanding & Overcoming Social Anxiety*. New York: Avon Books, 1996.

Social Anxiety Institute. http://www.socialanxietyinstitute.org/experiences.html.

The Social Anxiety Network International. http://www.anxietynetwork.com/sp.

Social Phobia/Social Anxiety Association. www.socialphobia.org.home.html.

Virtually Better. http://www.virtuallybetter.com.

Zoloft. http://www.zoloft.com/zoloft.portal?_nfpb = true&_pageLabel = default_home.

Index

Picture Credits

Biographies

Author

Joyce Libal is a writer and editor living in northeastern Pennsylvania. She has written numerous educational books including *Antidepressants and Suicide: When Treatment Kills, Drug Therapy and Substance-Related Disorders*, and *Drug Therapy for Mental Disorders Due to a Medical Condition.*

Consultant

Andrew M. Kleiman, M.D., received a Bachelor of Arts degree in philosophy from the University of Michigan, and earned his medical degree from Tulane University School of Medicine. Dr. Kleiman completed his internship, residency in psychiatry, and fellowship in forensic psychiatry at New York University and Bellevue Hospital. He is currently in private practice in Manhattan, specializing in psychopharmacology, psychotherapy, and forensic psychiatry. He also teaches clinical psychology at the New York University School of Medicine.